PHILADELPHIA

PHILADELPHIA • SUBURBS
SOUTH JERSEY • JERSEY SHORE
ATLANTIC CITY • DELAWARE

ROMAC REPORT

•1996•

ROMAC REPORT
P.O. Box 328
Villanova, PA 19085

610-519-0600

Published By

ROMAC REPORT
P.O. Box 328
Villanova, PA 19085

ISBN 0-9644383-2-1

CONTENTS

INTRODUCTION

This guide is the result of more than six months of intensive research, including a public opinion poll we conducted over the summer.

We asked residents of the Delaware Valley to give us their opinions on area restaurants they visited in the past year. More than 1,300 local frequent diners responded, providing us with over 60,000 numerical ratings, and hundreds of pages of commentary.

We started this project looking for local, inside information on Philadelphia area, South Jersey and Delaware restaurants. While we think our participants have provided us with the most accurate, up-to-date information available on the local dining scene, based on more meals than any single reviewer could ever eat, that is not the most impressive aspect of the poll. We were again most pleased with the rigor of our participants' work. The countless wrinkles, coffee stains, dog-ears and other signs of wear on the questionnaires indicate that our Romac Reporters spent many hours helping to make this book a success. We thank them heartily!

We also thank our writers and copyreader, who distilled the thousands of pages of material given us by our participants and the restaurants. Our writers are Andrew McElfresh, Joan M. Lang, and Al Mascitti. Our copyreader is Sarah McElfresh.

The ratings in this guide, while representing many thousands of votes, are subjective. We decided to represent ratings graphically, so readers can compare them at a glance. Most of the food ratings in this guide are "good" or better. While we went to the time and expense of rating over three times the number of restaurants that made it into the book, we included only restaurants our reviewers had reasons to recommend.

Finally, we owe a debt of gratitude to the restaurants. Despite the hard work and devotion they put into running their restaurants, most owners and managers took the time to answer our questions.

We urge you to find those places we may have overlooked. Be adventurous diners, and discover all the great restaurants across the Delaware Valley. Above all, let us know if there are any ways you think we can improve upon this guide. By the time next summer rolls around, you will be ready to participate in the '97 poll. In exchange for your efforts, you will receive a free copy of the 1997 Romac Report.

To participate in the 1997 poll, provide your name and address to us at one of the addresses or numbers below:

Romac Report '97, Philadelphia
P.O. Box 328
Villanova, PA 19085

Fax: (610) 519-0601

E-mail: RomacRpt@AOL.com

Bon appetit!

Charles W. McElfresh
Lynne V. Rosen

Rosemont, PA
November 6, 1995

PREFACE

What is the trend in Philadelphia these days? In with the casual—the trattoria, cafe, and bistro. Dress down, not up, and eat healthy.

So it is, in this ex-land of the blue blazer, that only 17 out of over 825 restaurants in our book require men to wear a jacket at dinner. Ask, as we did, all the restaurant owners and managers, "Describe your restaurant's atmosphere," and they will likely include the phrase "upscale casual" in their answers.

The Baby Boomers, now solidly into their peak restaurant-going years, are driving this trend. Why? Because they're also solidly into their family years, and, often, both parents have careers. Work-weary people would rather put the suit in the closet, rather than on, before they go out to eat. (No problem there, say younger folk.)

It's also because people want their meals out to be more like a regular meal and less like an event, because the trend toward a more casual atmosphere goes hand in hand with a trend toward lighter cuisine. Not many want to eat a big piece of meat at dinner anymore. What they really want is a smaller portion of chicken, meat, or fish, a big bowl of pasta, or rice or other grain, and a side of grilled vegetables.

Don't get us wrong: There are still plenty of big-night-out places. Start at Walnut Street, now the solid hub of the Philadelphia dining scene, and point your car in any direction. There are scores of formal restaurants, and wonderful, lovingly restored inns all over the Delaware Valley, which still have the big American, Continental and French menus and the big wines. If anything, the new trend toward lighter dining will help narrow this already competitive field.

Whatever drives the trend toward lighter, more casual dining, it is good news for Philadelphia. Many here have been eating this way their whole lives. That plate of fresh pasta you ordered, with a side of greens? It's been on the menu for years at a score of South Philly Italian restaurants. That fish or lobster, plucked fresh from the tank? Nothing new there, say a dozen Chinatown spots. Brick oven pizza wasn't invented yesterday, and rotisserie cooking has been around since fire was discovered.

The message is, then, don't just focus on the new places, but rediscover the old. Go to those restaurants you haven't visited for a while, and eat from the side of the menu you used to ignore.

And, most of all, enjoy!

Lynne V. Rosen
Charles W. McElfresh
Andrew J. McElfresh

Rosemont, PA
November 6, 1995

KEY TO SYMBOLS

Our survey participants rated restaurants' food, room and ambiance, and staff. The following pictures represent these categories:

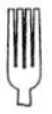 = Food

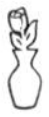 = Room and Ambiance

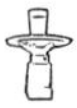 = Staff

Participants rated each restaurant's food, room and ambiance, and staff, on a scale of 0 (lowest) to 5 (highest). We averaged the scores, and converted them into the following bar graphs:

 = Superior

 = Excellent

 = Very Good

 = Good

 = Fair

= Poor

Survey participants also estimated the cost of one meal, with one drink and the tip. The average is printed after the ratings.

Where a restaurant either received too few votes to produce accurate ratings, or was new or written in by our voters, the ratings are replaced by the Romac Vote Box:

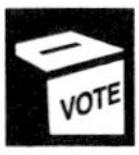

HOW TO USE THIS BOOK

The Romac Report is made up of three sections. The first section details the winners of various categories in our survey. The second section is the directory, which includes ratings and a review of each restaurant, along with its address and phone. The third section is made up of indexes, which list restaurant names and the page numbers for their directory listings. There are indexes for cuisine types, neighborhoods, and features.

There are three ways to use the Romac Report. First, start with the indexes, where you will find the cuisines and features you enjoy, in the neighborhoods where you plan to dine. Then, look up the reviews of those restaurants in the directory. Or, start with the first section, where you will find the restaurants our participants feel rate highest in several dozen categories; then find them in the directory. Finally, leaf through the directory and start reading—we think you'll enjoy it.

When you have chosen a restaurant, pick up the phone and call. Features, hours, reservation policies, even locations and cuisines change. When you return home, mark your scores in your book, and you'll be ready to participate in next year's Romac Report poll!

LEADERS of the POLL

Top 100 Favorites

1. Le Bec-Fin
2. Fountain
3. White Dog Cafe
4. Striped Bass
5. Dmitri's
6. Susanna Foo
7. Saloon
8. Jake's
9. Sonoma
10. Cafe Nola
11. Rose Tattoo Cafe
12. BLT's Cobblefish
13. Magnolia Cafe
14. Palm
15. Dilworthtown Inn
16. Ruth's Chris Steakhouse
17. Morton's of Chicago
18. Astral Plane
19. La Veranda
20. Ciboulette
21. Wild Orchid
22. Chart House
23. Zocalo
24. Le Bus Main St.
25. Friday, Saturday, Sunday
26. Outback Steakhouse
27. Garden
28. Zanzibar Blue
29. Judy's Cafe
30. Kansas City Prime
31. Pamplona
32. Nais Cuisine
33. Circa
34. Sagami
35. William Penn Inn
36. Toscana Cucina Rustica
37. Ralph's Italian
38. Deux Cheminees
39. Yangming
40. Stazi Milano
41. American Bistro
42. Cutter's
43. Reading Terminal Market
44. DiLullo Centro
45. Taquet
46. Mainland Inn
47. Primavera Pizza Kitchen
48. Bertucci's
49. Marabella's
50. Tira Misu
51. La Fourchette
52. Friday's
53. Braddock's Tavern
54. Passerelle
55. La Famiglia
56. Carolina's
57. Alisa Cafe
58. La Buca
59. Hikaru
60. Overtures
61. Bridgid's
62. Green Room
63. La Campagne
64. Under the Blue Moon
65. Blue Bell Inn
66. Upstares at Varalli
67. Old Original Bookbinders
68. Founders
69. London Grill
70. Central Bar & Grille
71. Grill & Bar
72. Genji I & II
73. Mustard Green
74. Napoleon Cafe
75. Aglio
76. Stephen's
77. Harry's Savoy Grill
78. Jack's Firehouse
79. Monte Carlo Living Room
80. Seven Stars Inn
81. Jefferson House
82. Dock Street Brewery
83. Griglia Toscana
84. Knave of Hearts
85. Houlihan's
86. Coventry Forge Inn
87. Rose Tree Inn
88. La Collina
89. Tree Tops
90. Meiji-En
91. Old Guard House Inn
92. Amara Cafe
93. Spring Mill Cafe
94. Copabanana/Copa Pronto
95. Adobe Cafe
96. Mrs. London's Cafe
97. Golden Pond Chinese
98. Alouette
99. Bunha Faun
100. Maureen

Top 50 Overall

1. Fountain
2. Le Bec-Fin
3. Green Room
4. Swann Lounge
5. Washington Inn
6. Grill & Bar
7. Deux Cheminees
8. Dining Room
9. Mainland Inn
10. Dilworthtown Inn
11. Brandywine Room
12. Striped Bass
13. Founders
14. Beau Rivage
15. La Campagne
16. Le Bar Lyonnais
17. La Truffe
18. Joe's
19. Mrs. London's Cafe
20. Frenchtown Inn
21. Ritz-Carlton Lobby Lounge
22. Ram's Head Inn
23. Morton's of Chicago
24. Back Burner
25. Sagami
26. Kamakura
27. Saloon
28. Braddock's Tavern
29. Cafe Gallery
30. Ciboulette
31. Susanna Foo
32. Coventry Forge Inn
33. Griglia Toscana
34. Monte Carlo Living Room
35. La Fourchette
36. Vickers Tavern
37. Phillips Mill, Inn at
38. Passerelle
39. Mendenhall Inn
40. Barrymore Room
41. La Bonne Auberge
42. Wild Orchid
43. Garden
44. Kimberton Inn
45. Marker
46. La Veranda
47. Siri's Thai French
48. Maureen
49. Yellow Springs Inn
50. Hamilton's Grill Room

Top 50 Food

1. Le Bec-Fin
2. Fountain
3. Sagami
4. Green Room
5. Le Bar Lyonnais
6. Wild Orchid
7. Carlino's
8. Joe's
9. Morton's of Chicago
10. Washington Inn
11. Swann Lounge
12. Mainland Inn
13. Dilworthtown Inn
14. Deux Cheminees
15. Dmitri's
16. White House Sub Shop
17. Griglia Toscana
18. Back Burner
19. American Bistro
20. Mrs. London's Cafe
21. Dining Room
22. Nais Cuisine
23. Grill & Bar
24. Susanna Foo
25. La Campagne
26. Striped Bass
27. Tacconelli's Pizza
28. Saloon
29. Alisa Cafe
30. Bunha Faun
31. La Truffe
32. Brandywine Room
33. Ciboulette
34. Frenchtown Inn
35. Vietnam
36. Rocco's Famous
37. Casselli's
38. Pink Rose Pastry Shop
39. Beau Rivage
40. Siri's Thai French
41. Coventry Forge Inn
42. Founders
43. Hamilton's Grill Room
44. BLT's Cobblefish
45. Zagara's
46. La Veranda
47. Jake's
48. Kansas City Prime
49. Ram's Head Inn
50. Palace of Asia

Top 50 Room & Ambiance

1. Fountain
2. Le Bec-Fin
3. Founders/Barrymore Room
4. Green Room
5. Striped Bass
6. Dining Room
7. Swann Lounge
8. Grill & Bar
9. Washington Inn
10. Deux Cheminees
11. Mansion on Main Street
12. Brandywine Room
13. Cafe Gallery
14. Phillips Mill, Inn at
15. Beau Rivage
16. Dilworthtown Inn
17. Ritz-Carlton Lobby Lounge
18. Kamakura
19. La Campagne
20. Planet Hollywood
21. Ram's Head Inn
22. Kennedy-Supplee Mansion
23. Victor Cafe
24. Mainland Inn
25. Tree Tops
26. Azalea at Omni Hotel
27. Cuttalossa Inn
28. Braddock's Tavern
29. Chateau Silvana
30. La Truffe
31. Yellow Springs Inn
32. Monte Carlo Living Room
33. Passerelle
34. La Bonne Auberge
35. Frenchtown Inn
36. Cousin's Country House
37. Vickers Tavern
38. Zanzibar Blue
39. Mendenhall Inn
40. Mrs. London's Cafe
41. Garden
42. Valley Green Inn
43. Kimberton Inn
44. Joseph Ambler Inn
45. Plumsteadville Inn
46. Rose Tattoo Cafe
47. Coventry Forge Inn
48. Primavera Pizza Kitchen
49. Duling-Kurtz
50. Ciboulette

Top 50 Staff

1. Fountain
2. Le Bec-Fin
3. Green Room
4. Swann Lounge
5. Washington Inn
6. Brandywine Room
7. Mainland Inn
8. Grill & Bar
9. Joe's
10. Beau Rivage
11. Deux Cheminees
12. Dilworthtown Inn
13. Ritz-Carlton Lobby Lounge
14. La Truffe
15. Dining Room
16. Victor Cafe
17. Founders
18. Frenchtown Inn
19. La Fourchette
20. Le Bar Lyonnais
21. Kamakura
22. Braddock's Tavern
23. Ram's Head Inn
24. Le Petit Cafe
25. La Campagne
26. Striped Bass
27. Mrs. London's Cafe
28. Saloon
29. Chanterelles
30. Griglia Toscana
31. Coventry Forge Inn
32. Cafe Gallery
33. Samuel's
34. Morton's of Chicago
35. Kimberton Inn
36. Passerelle
37. Abacus Chinese
38. Back Burner
39. Charles Plaza
40. La Bonne Auberge
41. Vickers Tavern
42. Mendenhall Inn
43. Loose Ends
44. Susanna Foo
45. Monte Carlo Living Room
46. Marker
47. Ciboulette
48. Marrakesh
49. Casselli's
50. Foggia

Top 25 Sleepers

1. Rib Crib
2. Green Hills Inn
3. Acacia
4. Gracie's 21st C. Cafe
5. Le Palais
6. Courtyard Cafe
7. Spiga D'Oro
8. Stockton Inn
9. Marriott's Seaview Resort
10. Carucci
11. Golden Pheasant Inn
12. Ebbit Room
13. Cafe Arielle
14. Cassatt Tea Room
15. Capriccio at Merv Griffin's
16. Filomena
17. Peter Shield's
18. Sweet Potato Cafe
19. Gourmet Restaurant
20. Jean-Pierre's
21. La Fourno
22. Volare
23. Pipersville Inn
24. Renault A'top the Winery
25. Tiffin

Top Food by Price

Top Food ($10 or less)

1. White House Sub Shop
2. Rocco's Famous
3. Pink Rose Pastry Shop
4. Tony Luke's
5. Fresh Fields Cafe
6. Jill's Vorspeise
7. Fairmount Bagel Institute
8. Dalessandro's Steaks
9. Sack O Subs
10. Jim's Steaks

Top Food ($11 to $20)

1. Carlino's Specialty Foods
2. Tacconelli's Pizza
3. Vietnam
4. Zagara's
5. Dardanelles
6. Abacus Chinese
7. Reading Terminal Market
8. Charles Plaza
9. Sampan Inn
10. Mama's Pizzeria

Top Food ($21 to $30)

1. Sagami
2. Wild Orchid
3. Dmitri's
4. Nais Cuisine
5. Bunha Faun
6. Caselli's
7. Siri's Thai French
8. BLT's Cobblefish
9. Palace of Asia
10. Giumarello's

TOPS BY CUISINE TYPES

Afghan
1. Kabul

American
1. Wild Orchid
2. Joe's
3. Morton's of Chicago
4. Washington Inn
5. Mainland Inn
6. Dilworthtown Inn
7. Back Burner
8. American Bistro
9. Dining Room
10. Grill & Bar

BBQ
1. Rib Crib
2. Rib Rack
3. Ron's Ribs
4. Broad Axe Tavern
5. Red, Hot & Blue

Belgian
1. Bridgid's

Brazilian
1. Brasil's

Burmese
1. Rangoon Burmese

Cajun/Creole
1. Cafe Nola
2. Magnolia Cafe

Californian
1. Planet Hollywood

Caribbean
1. 410 Bank Street

Cheesesteaks, Hoagies, Etc.
1. White House Sub Shop
2. Rocco's Famous
3. Mama's Pizzeria
4. Celebre's Pizzeria
5. Dalessandro's Steaks
6. Sack O Subs
7. Sun Valley Pizza Co.
8. Jim's Steaks
9. Geno's Steaks
10. Stoxy's Steaks

Chinese
1. Susanna Foo
2. Abacus Chinese
3. Charles Plaza
4. Mustard Green
5. Sampan Inn
6. Sang Kee
7. Tang-Yean
8. Yangming
9. Lee How Fook
10. Golden Pond Chinese

Coffeehouse
1. Napoleon Cafe
2. Painted Parrot Cafe
3. Old City Coffee
4. Capriccio

Continental
1. Fountain
2. Swann Lounge
3. Dilworthtown Inn
4. American Bistro
5. Dining Room
6. Brandywine Room
7. Founders
8. Ram's Head Inn
9. Vickers Tavern
10. Rose Tree Inn

Crabs
1. DiNardo's
2. Byrnes Tavern
3. DiNardo's
4. Crab Pot
5. Hardshell Cafe

Deli
1. Bruno's
2. Michael's Deli
3. Murray's Deli
4. Famous 4th St. Deli
5. Ben & Irv's Rest. & Deli

Desserts
1. Swann Lounge
2. Pink Rose Pastry Shop
3. Painted Parrot Cafe
4. Main-ly Desserts
5. More Than Just Ice Cream

English
1. Dickens Inn

European
1. Overtures
2. Cousin's
3. Cousin's Country House
4. Warsaw Cafe

French
1. Le Bec-Fin
2. Fountain
3. Green Room
4. Le Bar Lyonnais
5. Dilworthtown Inn
6. Deux Cheminees
7. Nais Cuisine
8. La Campagne
9. Alisa Cafe
10. Bunha Faun

German
1. Otto's Brauhaus

Greek
1. Athens Cafe

Indian
1. Palace of Asia
2. New Delhi Indian
3. Passage to India
4. Tandoor India

Indonesian
1. Singapore Kosher

International
1. Mrs. London's Cafe
2. Loose Ends
3. Braddock's Tavern
4. Yangming
5. Samuel's
6. Zanzibar Blue
7. Villa Strafford
8. Under the Blue Moon
9. Mama Ventura's
10. Herb Garden Cafe

Irish
1. Brittingham's Irish Pub

Israeli
1. Maccabeam

Italian
1. Carlino's Specialty Foods
2. Griglia Toscana
3. Saloon
4. Casselli's
5. La Veranda
6. Monte Carlo Living Room
7. Giumarello's
8. Joe Italiano's
9. La Famiglia
10. Totaro's

Jamaican
1. Jamaican Jerk Hut

Japanese
1. Sagami
2. Kamakura
3. Genji I & II
4. Shiroi Hana
5. Meiji-En

Lebanese
1. Cedar's

Light Fare
1. Fairmount Bagel Institute
2. More Than Just Ice Cream
3. Old City Coffee
4. Dean & DeLuca
5. Capriccio

Macrobiotic
1. Mary's

Malaysian
1. Singapore Kosher

Mediterranean
1. Dmitri's
2. Hamilton's Grill Room
3. Stephen's
4. Circa
5. Quissett

Mexican
1. Zocalo
2. Tequila's
3. 12th Street Cantina
4. Mexican Food Factory
5. Mexican Post

Middle Eastern
1. Al Kimah
2. Persian Grill
3. Alyan's
4. Cedar's
5. Al Dar

Morrocan
1. Fez Moroccan
2. Al Kimah
3. Marrakesh

Pizza
1. Tacconelli's Pizza
2. Mama's Pizzeria
3. Celebre's Pizzeria
4. Grotto Pizza
5. Sun Valley Pizza Co.
6. Marra's
7. Felicia's Pizza Kitchen
8. Primavera Pizza Kitchen
9. Rizzo's Italian
10. Pepper Mill

Portuguese
1. La Paella Tio Pepe

Seafood
1. Striped Bass
2. BLT's Cobblefish
3. Kansas City Prime
4. Library II
5. DiNardo's
6. Barnacle Ben's
7. Essene Cafe
8. Pattaya (fka Sweet Basil)
9. Colombia Hotel
10. Meiji-En

Southwestern
1. Tex Mex Connection

Spanish
1. Pamplona

Steakhouse
1. Morton's of Chicago
2. Kansas City Prime
3. Palm
4. Ruth's Chris Steakhouse
5. Library II

Taiwanese
1. Ray's Coffee Shop

Tavern Fare
1. Byrnes Tavern

Tea
1. Swann Lounge
2. Ritz-Carlton Lobby Lounge
3. Barrymore Room
4. Cassatt Tea Room

Tex-Mex
1. Tex Mex Connection
2. North Star Bar

Thai
1. Siri's Thai French
2. Thai Garden
3. Thai Singha House
4. Amara Cafe
5. Pattaya

Turkish
1. Dardanelles

Vegetarian
1. Essene Cafe
2. Jill's Vorspeise

Vietnamese
1. Vietnam
2. Saigon
3. Vietnam Palace
4. Vang Garden

TOPS BY AREAS

Philadelphia

Art Museum Area
1. Rose Tattoo Cafe
2. Bridgid's
3. London Grill
4. Jack's Firehouse
5. Cafe Flower Shop

Chestnut Hill/Mt. Airy
1. Umbria
2. Roller's
3. Under the Blue Moon
4. Pollo Rosso
5. Cafette

Chinatown
1. Vietnam
2. Charles Plaza
3. Sang Kee
4. Tang-Yean
5. Lee How Fook
6. Thai Garden
7. Ray's Coffee Shop
8. Golden Pond Chinese
9. Vietnam Palace
10. Joe's Peking Duck House

City Line Area
1. Marker
2. Bangkok Cuisine

Delaware Riverfront
1. La Veranda
2. Meiji-En
3. Chart House
4. Katmandu
5. Rock Lobster

Germantown
1. Ellen Rose

Historic Area
1. La Truffe
2. Dardanelles
3. La Famiglia
4. La Buca
5. Panorama
6. Kabul
7. Painted Parrot Cafe
8. Le Champignon
9. Azalea at Omni Hotel
10. Jeannine's Bistro

Manayunk/Roxborough
1. Casselli's
2. BLT's Cobblefish
3. Jake's
4. Kansas City Prime
5. Stephen's
6. Dalessandro's Steaks
7. Main-ly Desserts
8. Sonoma
9. Hikaru
10. Grasshopper

North Phila.
1. Tapas

Northeast Phila.
1. La Paella Tio Pepe
2. Moonstruck
3. Kawabata
4. La Padella
5. Stoxy's Steaks

Northern Liberties
1. Liberties
2. Ortleib's Jazz House

Port Richmond
1. Tacconelli's Pizza
2. Napoleon Cafe
3. Byrnes Tavern

South Phila.
1. Dmitri's
2. Saloon
3. Overtures
4. La Grolla
5. Saigon
6. Essene Cafe
7. Tony Luke's
8. Joseph's Italian
9. La Vigna
10. Celebre's Pizzeria

South Street Area

1. Pink Rose Pastry Shop
2. Monte Carlo Living Room
3. Mustard Green
4. Primavera
5. San Carlo
6. Tira Misu
7. Cafe Nola
8. Judy's Cafe
9. Alouette
10. Chef's Market

University City/West Phila.

1. White Dog Cafe
2. Genji I & II
3. Zocalo
4. Thai Singha House
5. Pattaya (fka Sweet Basil)
6. Lemon Grass Thai
7. New Delhi Indian
8. Restaurant School

Phila. Suburbs & Beyond

Berks County

1. Joe's

Bucks County

1. Phillips Mill, Inn at
2. La Bonne Auberge
3. Il Sol D'Italia
4. Plumsteadville Inn
5. Conti Cross Keys Inn

Chester County

1. Dilworthtown Inn
2. Vickers Tavern
3. Mendenhall Inn
4. Seven Stars Inn
5. Yellow Springs Inn

City Line Area

1. Alberto's
2. San Marco

Delaware County

1. American Bistro
2. Nais Cuisine
3. Alisa Cafe
4. Rose Tree Inn
5. Sampan Inn

Lancaster County

1. Donecker's

Main Line

1. Carlino's Specialty Foods
2. Bunha Faun
3. La Fourchette
4. Passerelle
5. Toscana Cucina Rustica

Montgomery County

1. Mainland Inn
2. Coventry Forge Inn
3. Palace of Asia
4. Abacus Chinese
5. Totaro's

New Jersey

Central Jersey

1. Acacia
2. Frenchtown Inn
3. Stockton Inn
4. Hamilton's Grill Room
5. Alchemist & Barrister

Jersey Shore

1. Washington Inn
2. White House Sub Shop
3. Le Palais
4. Marriott's Seaview Resort
5. Ram's Head Inn
6. Maureen
7. Ebbit Room
8. 410 Bank Street
9. Capriccio at Merv Griffin's
10. Frescos

South Jersey

1. Sagami
2. Wild Orchid
3. Mrs. London's Cafe
4. La Campagne
5. Beau Rivage
6. Siri's Thai French
7. Zagara's
8. Giumarello's
9. Loose Ends
10. Joe Italiano's

Delaware

1. Green Room
2. Griglia Toscana
3. Back Burner
4. Brandywine Room
5. Carucci

TOPS BY FEATURES

After Work Drink

1. Cutter's
2. Dock Street Brewery
3. Friday's
4. Fountain
5. Circa
6. Sonoma
7. Irish Pub
8. Houlihan's
9. Mace's Crossing
10. Sfuzzi

Bakeries

1. Le Bus
   Albrecht's Market
   Narberth
   (610) 667-7443
   on the Main Line
   Reading Terminal Market
   11th & Filbert Sts.
   Philadelphia
   (215) 592-0422
   in Center City
   220 Krams Ave.
   Philadelphia
   (215) 930-0255
   in Manayunk/Roxborough
2. Pink Rose Pastry Shop
3. Metropolitan Bakery
   262 S. 19th St.
   Philadelphia
   (215) 545-6655
   in Center City
   & other locations
4. Termini Bakery
   1523 S. 8th St.Philadelphia
   (215) 334-1816
   in So. Phila.
   & other locations
5. Baker Street
   316 S. 5th St.
   Philadelphia
   (215) 925-6620
   in the Historic Area
   & other locations
6. Viking Pastries
   39 Cricket Ave.
   Ardmore PA
   (610) 642-9227
   on the Main Line
7. Classic Cake Co.
   2028 Springdale Rd.
   Cherry Hill NJ
   (609) 751-5448
   in So. Jersey
8. Bredenbeck's Bakery
   8126 Germantown Ave.
   Philadelphia
   (215) 247-7374
   in Chestnut Hill/Mt. Airy
9. Reading Terminal Market
   12th & Filbert Sts.
   Philadelphia
   in Center City/Chinatown
10. Rindlaub's
    128 S. 18th St.
    Philadelphia
    (215) 563-3993
    in Center City

Bar Food

1. Friday's
2. Houlihan's
3. White Dog Cafe
4. Dock Street Brewery
5. Le Bar Lyonnais
6. Cutter's
7. Copabanana/Copa Pronto
8. Bridgid's
9. Dave & Buster's
10. London Grill

Barbecue

1. Rib-It
2. Red, Hot & Blue
3. Ron's Ribs
4. Rib Rack
5. Rib Crib
6. Manny Brown's
7. Broad Axe Tavern
8. Outback Steakhouse
9. Phoebe's
   2214 South St.
   Philadelphia
   (215) 546-4811
   in S.W. Phila.
10. Hickory Pit
    North Wales Train Station
    North Wales PA
    (215) 699-0590
    in Montgomery County

Brunch

1. Fountain
2. Meiji-En
3. Cafe Nola
4. Le Bus Main St.
5. Marker
6. Green Room
7. White Dog Cafe
8. William Penn Inn
9. Dining Room
10. Chart House

Business Dinner

1. Striped Bass
2. Palm
3. Morton's of Chicago
4. Fountain
5. Ruth's Chris Steakhouse
6. Susanna Foo
7. Cutter's
8. Garden
9. Le Bec-Fin
10. Kansas City Prime

Business Lunch

1. Palm
2. Fountain
3. Striped Bass
4. Cutter's
5. Sfuzzi
6. Le Bec-Fin
7. Morton's of Chicago
8. Marabella's
9. Circa
10. White Dog Cafe

Cheesesteak

1. Jim's Steaks
2. Pat's King of Steaks
3. Geno's Steaks
4. Dalessandro's Steaks
5. Mama's Pizzeria
6. Lee's Hoagies
7. Tony Luke's
8. Abner's
   3813 Chestnut St.
   Philadelphia
   (215) 662-0100
   in University City/W. Phila.
9. White House Sub Shop
10. Pepper Mill

Children

1. Dave & Buster's
2. Chuck E. Cheese
   9175 Roosevelt Blvd.
   Philadelphia
   (215) 677-6300
   in Northeast Phila.
   & other locations
3. Friday's
4. Bertucci's
5. Ground Round
   11295 Roosevelt Blvd.
   Philadelphia
   (215) 969-5334
   in Northeast Phila.
   & other locations
6. Al E. Gator's
7. Le Bus Main St.
8. McDonalds
   Many locations
9. Nifty Fifties
10. Spaghetti Warehouse

Coffeehouses

1. Dean & DeLuca
2. Ray's Coffee Shop
3. Barnes & Noble
   720 Lancaster Ave.
   Bryn Mawr PA
   (610) 520-0355
   on the Main Line
   & other locations
4. Starbuck's
   1528 Walnut Street
   Philadelphia
   (215) 732-0708
   in Center City
   & other locations
5. Last Drop Coffeehouse
6. Millenium Coffee
   212 S. 12th St.
   Philadelphia
   (215) 731-9798
   in Center City
7. Borders Books
   1727 Walnut St.
   Philadelphia
   (215) 568-7400
   in Center City
   & other locations
8. Old City Coffee
9. La Colombe
   130 S. 19th St.
   Philadelphia
   (215) 563-0860
   in Center City
   & other locations
10. Napoleon Cafe

Conversation

1. Sonoma
2. Fountain
3. White Dog Cafe
4. Borders Books
   1727 Walnut St.
   Philadelphia
   (215) 568-7400
   in Center City
   & other locations
5. Friday, Saturday, Sunday
6. Carolina's
7. Astral Plane
8. Le Bec-Fin
9. Rose Tattoo Cafe
10. Magnolia Cafe

Crabs

1. DiNardo's
2. Walt's
3. Hardshell Cafe
4. DiNardo's
5. Chickie & Pete's Cafe
   4010 Robbins Ave.
   Philadelphia
   (215) 338-1190
   in Northeast Phila.

Dessert

1. Le Bec-Fin
2. Napoleon Cafe
3. Main-ly Desserts
4. Painted Parrot Cafe
5. Pink Rose Pastry Shop
6. Fountain
7. White Dog Cafe
8. More Than Just Ice Cream
9. Jake's
10. Rose Tattoo Cafe

Diners

1. Melrose Diner
2. Ponzio's Kingsway
3. American Diner
4. Minella's
5. Diner on the Square
   1839 Spruce St.
   Philadelphia
   (215) 735-5787
   in Center City
6. Down Home Diner
7. Mayfair Diner
8. Country Club
9. Mastoris Diner
10. Country Squire Diner

Dives

1. Dirty Frank's
   347 S. 13th St.
   Philadelphia
   (215) 732-5010
   in Center City
2. McGlinchey's
   259 S. 15th St.
   Philadelphia
   (215) 735-1259
   in Center City
3. Triangle Tavern
4. Doobie's
   2201 Lombard St.
   Philadelphia
   (215) 546-0316
   in Center City
5. Strolli's
6. Copabanana
7. Walt's
8. Joe's Peking Duck House
9. Cherry Street Tavern
   129 N. 22nd St.
   Philadelphia
   (215) 561-5683
   in Center City
10. Sugar Mom's

Eavesdropping

1. Palm
2. Sonoma
3. Striped Bass
4. Cutter's
5. Le Bec-Fin
6. Borders Books
   1727 Walnut St.
   Philadelphia
   (215) 568-7400
   in Center City
7. Fountain
8. Kansas City Prime
9. Reading Terminal Market
10. Friday's

Espresso/Cappuccino

1. Dean & DeLuca
2. Borders Books
   1727 Walnut St.
   Philadelphia
   (215) 568-7400
   in Center City
   & other locations
3. Starbuck's
   1528 Walnut Street
   Philadelphia
   (215) 732-0708
   in Center City
   & other locations
4. Barnes & Noble
   720 Lancaster Ave.
   Bryn Mawr PA
   (610) 520-0355
   on the Main Line
   & other locations
5. Napoleon Cafe
6. La Colombe
   130 S. 19th St.
   Philadelphia
   (215) 563-0860
   in Center City
7. Millenium Coffee
   212 S. 12th St.
   Philadelphia
   (215) 731-9798
   in Center City
8. New World Cafe
   1625 Chestnut St.
   Liberty Place
   Philadelphia
   (215) 587-9230
   in Center City
   & other locations
9. Old City Coffee
10. Bucks County Coffee Co.
    many locations

Gay/Lesbian

1. Judy's Cafe
2. Woody's
   202 S. 13th St.
   Philadelphia
   (215) 545-1893
   in Center City
3. The Harmony Zone'
   254 S. 12th St.
   Philadelphia
   (215) 545-8088
   in Center City
4. Millenium Coffee
   212 S. 12th St.
   Philadelphia
   (215) 731-9798
   in Center City
5. Astral Plane

Live Entertainment

1. Zanzibar Blue
2. North Star Bar
3. Rock Lobster
4. Serrano/Tin Angel
5. Ortleib's Jazz House
6. Blue Moon Jazz
7. Katmandu
8. Victor Cafe
9. Grape Street Pub
   105 Grape St.
   Philadelphia
   (215) 483-4890
   in Manayunk/Roxborough
10. Triangle Tavern

Older Adults

1. Blue Bell Inn
2. Fountain
3. Williamson Restaurant
4. Little Pete's
5. Monte Carlo Living Room

Outdoor Dining

1. Garden
2. Rock Lobster
3. Katmandu
4. River Deck Cafe
5. Rosebud's Cafe
6. Jon's Bar & Grill
7. Sonoma
8. Cuttalossa Inn
9. Valley Green Inn
10. Bridget Foy's

Pizza

1. Tacconelli's Pizza
2. Bertucci's
3. Pizzeria Uno
   511 S. 2nd St.
   Philadelphia (215)
   592-0400
   in the Historic Area
4. Rizzo's Italian
5. Pizza Hut
   865 W. Lancaster Ave.
   Bryn Mawr PA
   (610) 527-5312
   on the Main Line
6. Mom's Bake at Home
   4452-54 Main St.
   Philadlephia PA
   (215) 487-2440
   in Manayunk/Roxborough
   & other locations
7. Marra's
8. Boccie Pizza
9. Sun Valley Pizza Co.
10. Grotto Pizza

Pre-Vet, Spectrum

1. Philly Rock Bar & Grill
2. Pat's King of Steaks
3. Celebre's Pizzeria
4. Marra's
5. Villa Di Roma
6. Tony Luke's
7. Melrose Diner
8. Ralph's Italian
9. Medora's Mecca
10. B. Criniti

Salad

1. Chart House
2. Saladalley
3. Olive Garden
   83 City Line Ave.
   Philadelphia
   (215) 664-4720
   in the City Line Area
4. Marathon Grill
5. Knave of Hearts
6. Sonoma
7. Le Bus Main St.
8. Judy's Cafe
9. Salad Works Cafe
   4700 City Line Ave.
   Philadelphia
   (215) 477-2121
   in the City Line Area
10. Frankie's Seafood Italiano

Singles Pickups

1. Cutter's
2. River Deck Cafe
3. Rock Lobster
4. Sonoma
5. Katmandu
6. Circa
7. Egypt Night Club
   520 N. Delaware Ave.
   Philadelphia
   (215) 922-6500
   on the Delaware Riverfront
8. Maui
   Pier 53, N. Delaware Ave.
   Philadelphia
   (215) 423-8116
   on the Delaware Riverfront
9. Carolina's
10. Irish Pub

Vegetarian menu

1. Mary's
2. Essene Cafe
3. Harmony Vegetarian
4. Charles Plaza
5. Cherry Street Chin. Veg.
6. Singapore Kosher
7. Golden Pond Chinese
8. Le Bus Main St.
9. Tang-Yean
10. Friday's

Views

1. Chart House
2. Meiji-En
3. Founders/Barrymore Rm.
4. Tree Tops
5. Fountain
6. Pyramid Club
   1735 Market St.
   Philadelphia
   (215) 567-6510
   in Center City
7. Rock Lobster
8. Valley Green Inn
9. La Veranda
10. Spirit of Philadelphia

Wine List

1. Le Bec-Fin
2. Panorama
3. Fountain
4. Dilworthtown Inn
5. La Famiglia
6. Abbey Wine Bar
7. Kansas City Prime
8. Zanzibar Blue
9. Striped Bass
10. White Dog Cafe

DIRECTORY

OF

RESTAURANTS

Philadelphia Area

Abacus Chinese

$20

1551 Valley Forge Rd., North Penn Market Place, Lansdale (215) 362-2010 at Sumneytown Pk. in Montgomery County

"Who would have thought a great Chinese would be in a strip shopping center in Lansdale?" Well, it turns out, just about everybody who has ever been to this "wonderful," "fresh," and even "inspiring" Szechuan in the North Penn Market Place. "The Maitre d' is a card," and "the staff is WONDERFUL." The cool fish tank ("more interesting than the Camden Aquarium") and Chinese music give this place an above-average room and ambiance rating. Don't forget the Chinese pizza at what many consider to be the "best Chinese in the 'burbs."

Abbey Wine Bar at the Radnor Hotel

$27

591 E. Lancaster Ave., St. Davids (610) 341-3165 at Radnor-Chester Rd. on the Main Line

A big, airy dining room overlooking a formal garden, nightly entertainment, and a well-received wine list make this Regional American in St. Davids' hopping Radnor Hotel a hit with the Main Line older singles crowd. Some survey participants applaud recent menu changes; others say the food "doesn't live up to the menu description."

Abyssinia (fka Red Sea)

VOTE

229 S. 45th St., Philadelphia (215) 387-2424 at Locust St. in University City/W. Phila.

Some folks think the Red Sea parted, but actually they just changed the name, and did a cursory renovation to this University City Ethiopian. Most diners think the "most unusual food" deserves pretty good marks, though the setting is one of the city's least appealing. Remembering that Ethiopian spices are not to everyone's taste, our voters recommend it for more adventurous palates.

Adobe Cafe

$19

4550 Mitchell St., Philadelphia (215) 483-3947 bet. Krams & Leverington in Manayunk/Roxborough

The so-so ratings for this popular Manayunk Mexican have our voters playing it safe: stick to simple food like "great wings and steak tips," but be prepared to wait, it "seems to be understaffed," with "slow but friendly service." While some aspects of the Adobe may be "going downhill," the place is still very child-friendly, and the "lively atmosphere" appeals to all age groups.

Adrienne's Bistro

$29

530 South St., Philadelphia (215) 829-9620 bet. 5th & 6th in the South St. Area

Pipe and cigar smokers will find a tiny refuge in one part of the bar at this Society Hill French, American and Californian bistro, but not much else. The "cozy" atmosphere does little better than the food, and our voters advise you to keep it simple when ordering. One reviewer notes, "Ralph the bartender has a special drink for every occasion." We hear he serves them, too.

 = Superior = Excellent = Very Good

Aglio

$36

937 E. Passyunk Ave., Philadelphia (215) 336-8008
bet. 6th & 7th & Carpenter in So. Phila.

This casual but style-conscious South Philly New Generation Italian scores highest with the 31-45 set, who best appreciate its "chic ambiance," "good bar," "stellar staff," and "imaginative, Italian-based cuisine." Garlic is the star (roasted garlic soup is a signature dish), but Romac Reporters also praise the gnocchi, pasta and veal chops. All this has made it hard to snag a seat in the small room, perhaps one reason the staff comes in for criticism among older voters.

Alberto's

$36

1415 City Ave., Wynnewood (610) 896-0275
Haverford & City Aves. in the City Line Area

This "first-class" Northern Italian in Wynnewood keeps regulars so happy with homemade pasta, double-cut veal chops and fresh fish dishes that they'll tolerate service even fans say is slow. Don't miss the agnolotti, half-moon-shaped pasta stuffed with spinach, ricotta and Parmesan.

Alberto's Newtown Squire

$35

191 S. Newtown Street Rd., Newtown Square (610) 356-9700
in Delaware County

With the same owners as Alberto's, Villa Strafford, and La Collina, the emphasis at this Italian and American restaurant in Newtown Square is on the decor, though the food could use more attention, according to voters. But what a setting—situated on 4 acres, with a natural pond, the decor features imported tiles, granite and ceramics from Italy. While some feel the food is "excellent," most call it "overpriced," and something of a "disappointment."

Al Dar

$21

281 Montgomery Ave., Bala Cynwyd (610) 667-1245
Old Lancaster & Levering Mill Rds. on the Main Line

"Variety comes to the suburbs" in the form of this Bala Cynwyd Middle Eastern. Decibel-challenged voters warn it "can be noisy," but say that it's worth it for the "excellent dishes" and the "best warm pita bread." Fans appreciate the wine by the glass and an interesting chicken Caesar salad. If you've tried it before, you may want to take a second look.

Al E. Gator's

$18

625 Lancaster Ave., Haverford (610) 525-5577
on the Main Line
260 W. Swedesford Rd., Berwyn (610) 640-4000
on the Main Line

As far as Romac Reporters are concerned, there's not much difference between a gator and a crock. This Main Line American trolls the same waters as Bennigan's, Houlihan's and their ilk, with a little more emphasis on families with kids. Some say it's a "fun place for children," although one warns "the alligator wouldn't sign my nephew an autograph." "Stay with the bar food"—the rest of the menu got hammered by voters, who say "they need to clean up their act."

= Good — = Fair [no rating] = Poor

FOOD ROOM STAFF COST

Alexander's

$22

1482 York Rd., Abington (215) 576-9766
at Wheatsheaf Rd. in Montgomery County

While this Abington restaurant purports to serve "Continental food with a Greek flair," our voters recommend that you stick to the "good, authentic Greek dishes." Whatever the meal, you get "large portions" that are "freshly prepared." Romac Reporters appreciate its many features, from ample parking to good desserts, in a kid-friendly atmosphere. Alexander's even has two fireplaces—but ask before you start throwing your plates.

Alfio's

$24

15 Limekiln Pk., Glenside (215) 885-3787
bet. Mt. Carmel & Willow Grove in Montgomery County

This Glenside Italian-American is aptly named—patrons come for tableside preparations of classic Caesar salad and sinful coffee romantico "made by Alfio the magician." That's not just a figure of speech—the owner also amuses customers with "fun coin and card tricks."

Alfonso's

$15

7232 Haverford Ave., Phila. (215) 473-3441 in the City Line Area

This Overbrook Italian is one of the most kid-friendly spots in the area: it has a kid's menu, and welcomes parents with infants. A low cost, "wonderful family Italian restaurant," the food is "basic," but "good." When the owner says to "bring the kids and their pictures and we'll hang them"—we assume he means the pictures.

Alisa Café

$31

109 Fairfield Ave., Upper Darby (610) 352-4402 in Del. County

In the top 30 for food, and one of Philadelphia's favorites, this teeny Upper Darby spot has been serving "excellent," "delicious" French food with Oriental influences to satisfied diners, Tuesday through Saturday for twelve years now. The "superb food" at reasonable prices plus a BYOB policy make this "out of the way place" a real find.

Alouette

$38

334 Bainbridge St., Philadelphia (215) 629-1126
at 4th St. in the South St. Area

What is a "wonderful Thai influence" to some does not appeal to everyone at this South Street Area French. Still, many voters give it top ratings for food, saying it's "consistently perfect in both preparation and presentation," though "pricey." Either way, it is a "very romantic" spot, in an historic setting, with great desserts and plenty of wines by the glass. There's even a place for pipe and cigar smokers.

Alpha Pizza House

$14

Haverford Ave. & Drexel Rd., Philadelphia (215) 473-6200
in the City Line Area

Families flock to this City Line neighborhood spot for the friendly atmosphere, big portions, and the kitchen's signature dishes, garlic chicken and an antipasto-style house salad.

Alyan's

$11

603 S. 4th St., Philadelphia (215) 922-3553
at South St. in the South St. Area

Arabic music and decor set the mood at this Middle Eastern "cheap eats oasis" on South Street. Many voters think it's a "hole in the wall," but they rave about the "inexpensive, tasty food," especially the charcoal-grilled meats. There's also plenty for vegetarians to choose from, and parents say the management is "nice to kids." BYO.

Amara Cafe

$21

105 S. 22nd St., Philadelphia (215) 564-6976
bet. Sansom & Chestnut in Center City

Fresh local ingredients and a major effort from the staff prove a winning combination at this tiny downtown Thai. While a room with only 30 seats might be "too small" for some with "tables too close together," owner Wallapa Phutlek more than makes up for it with "very good Thai food, prepared with imagination." Few seats, great food and lunch specials pack the place, making reservations essential. The "incredible wing bean salad" is a perennial favorite.

American Bistro

$36

Rt. 420 & Morton Ave., Morton (610) 543-3033
in Delaware County

The location "does nothing for this restaurant" and patrons must bring their own wine, but Romac Reporters call this Regional American "Delco's Le Bec-Fin" and rank it among the top 20 for food. Owner-chef James Webb's "unique and sensual" cuisine, featuring exotic meats and lots of fruit, are "special combinations—no two are alike." Voters praise the staff, but grouse that there's "no ambiance," and a few gripe about the prices. The consensus: "worth the trip—but call well in advance."

American Diner

$11

42nd & Chestnut Sts., Philadelphia (215) 387-1451
in University City

Third on our Top 10 list of diners, our voters tell us it's "great for pie and coffee, late at night." Well, it is a DINER, after all. A recent change of hands has made some voters doubt this University City American, but we think another visit for "the best waffles and pancakes" might bring them back into the fold.

Appleby's at the Adams Mark

$18

City Ave. & Monument Rd., Philadelphia (215) 581-5000
in the City Line Area

"Not your typical hotel coffee shop" say voters of this American restaurant, set in the Adam's Mark hotel on City Line Avenue. While the overall food rating is pretty low, the comments suggest you don't simply pass it by: "try their early bird specials," suggests one, though they may be strictly "non-gourmet." The simple pleasures, like "fast, cheap food and good salads," make this "a good family restaurant."

FOOD ROOM STAFF COST

Archie's Tavern

$14

603 Summit Ave., Jenkintown (215) 576-9154
at Rt. 611 in Montgomery County

"Every neighborhood needs a good local bar with good food," one Romac Reporter notes. In Jenkintown, they have Archie's. The food is just fair, but prices are low.

Arizona Cafe

$18

1543 Spring Garden St., Philadelphia (215) 567-5555
at 16th St. in the Art Museum Area

"Why oh why is it no longer open for dinner?" laments one reviewer of this Art Museum-area Southwestern restaurant. What they do is lunch only, weekdays only, and they do it right, with good ratings for simple, well prepared food with many Jefferson Dining With Heart items. There's also an outdoor cafe in season.

Artful Dodger

$19

4th & Pine Sts., Philadelphia (215) 922-7880 in the Historic Area

A large sample of voters deem the American/Continental pub fare at this little Historic Area spot fair-to-middlin'. We think it may be the closest thing to the pubs of our forefathers: Pipes and cigars are welcome at the bar, there's live entertainment on weekends, darts all the time, and although the food is unexciting, "the drinking is better."

Arts Bank Cafe (fka Café des Artistes)

$20

Broad & South Sts., Phila. (215) 545-4580 in the South St. Area

Management says it's "redefining the basic idea of the arts cafe" with performance events every night ranging from music to poetry and dance. Voters say they should redefine the American light fare, which gets only fair ratings, and get rid of the "sometimes surly" service.

Asakura

$28

339 N. Lansdowne Ave., Lansdowne (610) 259-4052 in Del. County

The owners of Le Champignon and Asa Cafe have a winner in this Landsdown Japanese restaurant. The food is "very good," with "excellent sushi and great service (I tip well here)." Voters recommend the tatami room, "where you sit on the floor and eat at a Japanese table." A BYO policy keeps prices down, while a separate no smoking room keeps sensitive diners happy.

Astral Plane

$30

1708 Lombard St., Phila. (215) 546-6230 (17th St. in Ctr City)

The funky, objet-filled room's the thing at this mid-priced Center City Modern American, a '70s holdover that for regulars is "an old standard, like a favorite song." The "clever atmosphere without being too cute" makes it a "great date restaurant" and "a special place for special times"; the unisex, black bathroom is an attention-grabber. But while some praise the "splendid soups," a few longtimers say the food has become "appallingly bland," and, although there is a no-smoking section, the "very smoky" room is "the only negative to an otherwise fine restaurant."

= Superior = Excellent = Very Good

Athena

$27

264 Keswick Ave., Glenside (215) 884-1777 (in Montgomery Cty.)
BYO and eat indoors or outdoors at this Glenside spot, where the Greek food is made from old family recipes. Voters praise the homemade hummus and pita bread. Prices are reasonable.

Azalea at Omni Hotel

$38

401 Chestnut St., Phila. (215) 931-4260 (at 4th St. in Historic Area)
All agree the view of Independence Park and the "beautiful room" are the highlights of this Historic Area American. "It's all downhill from there," say some, but others think the food is fine, especially at the "great Sunday brunch."

Baci Bistro

$23

211 S. Broad St., Philadelphia (215) 731-0700
at Walnut St. in Center City
The bar scene draws the crowd at this Center City Modern Italian. The bi-level dining room overlooks the bar, decorated with a romantic theme. The food's "innovative, unusual combinations" earn only fair grades, but the cruvinet machine with fine wines by the glass make it "great for a drink after the orchestra."

Bailey's

$16

1280 Whiteland Town Ctr., Exton (610) 524-2424 Rts. 30 & 100
on the Main Line
This casual American in Exton is not really the "come for the food" kind of place. While the food may be "good," with the "best sandwiches" and "big portions" standouts, you won't find anything memorable on the menu. Our voters do remember Bailey's fondly as a fun nightclub, with live rock bands and dancing on weekend evenings.

Balligo Inn

$22

16 Balligomingo Rd., Gulph Mills (610) 828-5615 in Mont. County
The poor ratings don't tell the whole story at this Gulf Mills restaurant, which serves the most rudimentary fare. Live Jazz on Saturday is why Romac Reporters go. The great selection of imported beers doesn't hurt, either.

Baltimore Junction Cafe

VOTE

242 W. Baltimore Pk., Clifton Heights (610) 259-6600
at Oak Ave. in Delaware County
The American and Italian fare, though no great innovation at this Clifton Heights yearling, is recommended by the few Romac Reporters who have visited this cafe. That's good news, since many restaurants that have murder mystery nights put on the show to make up for a questionable kitchen. An "inexpensive" tab, a BYOB policy and the fact that "they really like kids," make it tough to find a reason not to stop at this junction.

FOOD ROOM STAFF COST

Bangkok Cuisine

$21

7552 Haverford Ave., Philadelphia (215) 877-1664
bet. City & Sherwood Aves. in the City Line Area

This City Line area spot is pricier than the typical Thai, though by no means expensive. The French-influenced, candlelit decor is also quite a bit classier, as the room rating shows. "Order the specials," which change weekly. The French touch also shows up on the wine list.

Barclay Dining Room at the Barclay Hotel

$33

On Rittenhouse Sq., Philadelphia (215) 545-0300 in Center City

Check out the Barclay dining room after November, when the restaurant will move back into the main dining room of this old Deco-era hotel. Room and ambiance ratings should climb then—we're hoping the same happens with the French cuisine.

Baron's Inne

$37

499 N. Gulph Rd., King of Prussia (610) 265-2550
in Montgomery County

This American-Continental in King of Prussia features a fireplace and live piano music for a "soothing atmosphere" that scores particularly well with middle-aged voters. It also offers wines by the glass and a heart-healthy menu. Reservations suggested.

Barrymore Room at the Bellevue Hotel

$38

Broad & Walnut, Philadelphia (215) 790-2814 (in Center City)

This cabaret in the Bellevue overlooking Center City is "a veritable pleasure dome." Enjoy the "graceful" setting and stunning view during December Nutcracker Tea, when local high school choirs sing. Says one Tory: "Look out the window with the most important person in your life" and you'll feel like "the King and Queen of Philadelphia."

Bassett's Original Turkey

$9

15th & Locust Sts., Philadelphia (215) 546-1812
in Center City & many other locations

Turkey lovers still flock to this Center City "healthy alternative to fast food" and its outlying branches, but it's starting to feel the competition—some say the "turkey has lost its gobble," and gripe about the price. Most still visit to experience "Thanksgiving all year."

Baxter's

$19

14 Paoli Shopping Ctr., Paoli (610) 296-2699
on the Main Line

The food may be only "fair" at this neighborhood American in Paoli, but there are other features that make up for it. There's a "good selection on the wine list," and at happy hour it's a "great place for complimentary hors d'oeuvres, from cheese to cold cuts and spreads." The concensus—"overpriced for location and quality of food."

 = Superior = Excellent = Very Good

Bay Pony Inn

$31

Old Skippack Rd.& Rt. 113, Lederach (215) 256-6565 in Mont. Co.

As in The Camptown Races, the Bay Pony is a good bet for "cozy, romantic" country dining. There are no surprises on the Continental menu, but the "sophisticated country setting" of this restored inn, with its fireplace and lovely meadow views, has many fans saying "take me to your Lederach." Early bird specials and banquet facilities are pluses.

Bay Street

$21

11000 Roosevelt Blvd., Phila. (215) 677-2370 in Northeast Phila.

Our voters usually find it easy to be unkind to chain restaurants. And while the numbers are consistent with that theory for this Northeast Philadelphia seafooder, the comments indicate a grudging approval. "The food is interesting—for a chain," writes one; another says it has "well prepared seafood at a decent price."

B. Criniti

$17

2601 S. Broad St., Phila. (215) 465-7750 at Shunk St. in So. Phila.

Traditional Italian food in "huge portions" keeps 'em coming to this homey, family-run spot in South Philly, convenient to the Vet and the Spectrum. The room is plain and small, so it's "crowded on weekends," but everything is homemade and you can bring your own beer and wine, adding up to an "extremely inexpensive" meal.

Beijing

$14

3714 Spruce St., Phila. (215) 222-5242 in Univ. City/W. Phila.

You get fresh Chinese food at a good price (due to high volume) at this University City spot. Though "they shuffle you in and out way too fast," you may well find "the best Chinese food outside of Chinatown." You can't reserve, and it's "always packed and noisy."

Bella Trattoria

$19

4258 Main St., Phila. (215) 482-5556 in Manayunk/Roxborough

Many voters give the food at this Manayunk BYO Italian their highest rating, but a few grumblers bring down the average. It may not be Italy, but it is "nice to sit outside" at a table on the Main Street sidewalk, eat the "inexpensive, quality food," and listen—on Fridays at least—to the accordianist, who plays Neapolitan songs. Order an espresso, and stay the evening.

Ben & Irv's Deli

$14

1962 County Line Rd., Justa Farm Shopping Center, Huntingdon Valley (215) 355-2000 in Montgomery County
Summit Sq. Shopping Ctr., Langhorne (215) 860-4601 in Bucks Co.

These New York style delis, so naturally voters think the service is "rude"—you got a problem with that? People will put up with "cramped seating" and other aggravations for a great corned beef special and "a good-time kosher experience." A few grumble about the price; more tout the "extremely generous portions." And nobody complains about the smoke-free environment.

FOOD ROOM STAFF COST

Bennigan's

$17

720 Baltimore Pk., Springfield (610) 328-0612 in Del. County
One Devon Sq., Devon (610) 964-1100 on the Main Line
King of Prussia Shopping Ctr., King of Prussia (610) 337-0633
Gulph Rd. & Rt. 202 in Montgomery County
2231 Cottman Ave., Philadelphia (215) 722-1902 in NE Phila.
11000 Roosevelt Blvd., Philadelphia (215) 677-4667 in NE Phila.
2402 Easton Rd., Willow Grove (215) 674-8383 in Mont. County

Even voters who gave this American pub chain good marks had little positive to say—"good drinks, but get out the Maalox" was typical. The many who slagged it were more forthcoming—"the dullest of dull food" in a "run-of-the-mill singles restaurant" sums it up.

Benny the Bum's

$23

9991 Bustleton Ave., Philadelphia (215) 673-3000
at Red Lion Rd. in Northeast Phila.

The name is only slightly more appetizing than the seafood dishes at this large, Northeast Philly family spot. Voters disagree strongly, with comments ranging from "awful" to "the best." From early bird specials to a well-known late menu, some voters are pickier than others.

Berlengas Island

$21

4926 N. 5th St., Philadelphia (215) 324-3240
2 Blks. off Roosevelt Blvd. in Northeast Phila.

While the room could use an overhaul, they still want you to dress up for this little North Philly "authentic" Portuguese, that some diners still consider "small and romantic." And while they have a very limited wine selection by the glass, voters advise that what starts as a low dining tab can climb up with drinks. P.S. Some think it's a "bad area at night."

Bertucci's

$17

1515 Locust St., Philadelphia (215) 731-1400
bet. 15th & 16th Sts. in Center City
2190 County Line Rd., The Marketplace, Huntingdon Valley
(215) 322-2200 (in Montgomery County)
675 Middletown Blvd., Oxford Valley Mall, Langhorne
(215) 752-9200 in Montgomery County
523 W. Lancaster Ave., Wayne (610) 293-1700 on the Main Line

The open kitchen with wood-burning stove sets the tone and pours out great pizza and dinner rolls at this chain, dubbed a "yuppie Pizza Hut" by some. Most agree the young, boisterous crowd, smoke-free atmosphere and "pleasant wait staff" make it a great spot for kids, who may play with raw pizza dough while they wait for their food. The pizza ranked No. 2 in the survey.

Between Friends at the Wyndham

$27

17th & Race Sts., Philadelphia (215) 448-2000 (in Center City)

The staff isn't between jobs at this Center City American/Continental restaurant; they are characterized as "very good" by our voters. So, too, are the "outstanding buffet lunch," and "delicious desserts," but when it comes to dinner there are few standouts. You must reserve ahead of time for the Sunday brunch, and our voters say it's worth it.

 = Superior = Excellent = Very Good

Beyond Measure

VOTE

1710 Sansom St., Phila. (215) 564-2000 at 17th St. in Center City
Bring the kids, a big appetite and your own wine or beer, if you choose, to this new "upscale, serve-yourself cafe." Sacrificing service for speed, without sacrificing quality of food, for very good Continental-based Eclectic fare, the price is right.

Bistro Bix

VOTE

114 S. 12th St., Phila. (215) 925-5336 bet. Chestnut & Sansom in Ctr. City
This grand cafe, taking over the lovely rooms of the old Odeon, is named after jazz great Bix Beiderbecke. It opened after our survey was completed, so Romac Reporters have not yet rated it. There's a jazz brunch on Sundays, $4 parking at 12th & Sansom, and plans for poetry readings and an art gallery on the third floor.

Bistro Perrier

VOTE

210 W. Rittenhouse Sq., The Rittenhouse, Phila. (215) 496-9605 in Center City
The trend today is away from the formal, big-night-out places, and toward the upscale casual, more-small-nights-out spots, where no jacket or tie is the rule, not the exception, and where the fare is simple and light. Case in point: Restaurant 210 closed, Georges Perrier takes over its space and teams up with Francesco Martonella, to create his version of the modern French bistro. The opening is planned for spring, 1996.

Bistro Romano

$24

120 Lombard St., Phila. (215) 925-8880 bet. Front & 2nd in the Historic Area
This "intimate," mid-priced Italian in Society Hill, located in a 200-year-old granary, presents "great tableside caesar salad" and plenty of heart-healthy options. Romac Reporters like the "warm, homey feel" of the "cozy booths" in the cool, stone grotto downstairs. The upstairs lounge features a piano bar on weekends.

Bistro San Tropez

$22

The Marketplace, 23rd & Market, Phila. (215) 569-9269 in Center City
We hear the "excellent French bistro" food at this good looking, and professionally staffed Center City restaurant is just perfect for "the ladies who lunch" crowd. While there is some talk of small portions, the low price tag, with prix fixes and other specials, still make it a good value, at this quality. The bonus at dinner is the lovely view of the Schuykill, and 30th Street Station across the river.

Black Bass Hotel

$39

3774 River Rd., Lumberville (215) 297-5770 in Bucks County
There's a chance this place has served more "charming and romantic" meals than any other in our book: it has been serving lunch and dinner since 1745. The "terrific view of the river" enhances the "great country setting," and only a few grumblers mar an otherwise excellent staff rating. In spite of its history, the American menu is in no way revolutionary, with one diner calling it "so-so at times."

FOOD ROOM STAFF COST

Black Walnut

VOTE

80 W. State St., Doylestown (215) 348-0708 in Bucks County
Jack Gudin, formerly of La Metairie in New York, just opened this tiny cafe in a cottage on State Street in Doylestown. Hardwood floors, a few antiques, and a lemon-yellow wash on the walls make for a simple country atmosphere. There's also a patio for when the weather's nice. Too new for our survey, this place looks promising. BYO, no credit cards.

BLT's Cobblefish

$27

443 Shurs Ln., Philadelphia (215) 483-5478
1 1/2 blocks below Ridge Ave. in Manayunk/Roxborough
This offbeat Manayunk Seafood restaurant, one of Romac Reporters' favorite places, aroused strong emotions—mostly raves—for the "creatively done fish," featuring more than a few "fish I never even heard of," all bought that morning. Voters enjoy it as "a funkier alternative to that other hip fish place," Striped Bass. The move to larger quarters has alleviated the chronic crowding, and prices are still reasonable thanks to the BYO policy.

Blue Bell Inn

$33

601 Skippack Pk., Blue Bell (215) 646-1576
at Pennlyn-Bluebell Pk. in Montgomery County
Many reviewers describe the Continental-American fare at this Montgomery County "landmark inn" as "geriatric dining," but it actually gets higher scores from middle-aged and younger voters. True, the decor, the piano music and dishes like chateaubriand and steak add up to "traditional food in a traditional setting," but many say that "in some 40 years this place has remained top-rate on all scores." And it has changed at least a little with the times—how else do you explain such dishes as blackened swordfish with pinapple rum sauce, or the special menu for the warm-weather outdoor cafe?

Blue Moon Jazz

$29

21 S. 4th St., Bourse Bldg., Philadelphia (215) 413-2272
bet. Market & Chestnut Sts. in the Historic Area
You'll find "great music for Jazz lovers," provided you don't mind paying a cover and can get yourself down to the Historic Area. And while you're looking at the menu, look twice—they have two distinctive menus in the two separate rooms: one room is a showcase with live jazz seven nights a week, the other a dining room with finer dining available. The "cool mixed ethnic scene" is overseen by "great" owners Ron Zaken and Sean Mann.

Boathouse Row Bar at the Rittenhouse Hotel

$17

210 W. Rittenhouse Sq., Phila. (215) 546-9000 (19th St. in Ctr. City)
You can't row a shell without bending your elbows, and that's exactly the attraction of this Center City pub. Most voters give the bar food fair grades but go for the atmosphere—a big mural of Boathouse Row along the Schuylkill, big-screen TVs and a good selection of frosty lagers.

Bobby's Seafood $26

5492 W. Chester Pk., Newtown Square (610) 296-4430
at Plumsock Rd. in Delaware County

With an "all-you-can-eat crab" selection, and what some call the "best oyster bar around," the buzz about this high-traffic, mid-sized seafooder in Newtown Square is a lot better than its ratings. Compare the middle-of-the-road votes with the bargain prix fixe lunch ($7.95) or dinner ($16.95), a good-looking, bustling crowd, and a casual, kid-friendly atmosphere, and it's no wonder voters call it "a good place to bring guests." Reservations essential.

Boccie $19

104 Coulter Ave., Suburban Sq., Ardmore (610) 658-0580
on the Main Line

This Main Line Italian/brick oven pizza joint is not connected to the Boccie in University City, and you can tell by the scores. The owners promise a renovation, but voters say the problems are "inconsistent food" and service that "needs some new help."

Boccie Pizza $15

4040 Locust St., The Warehouse, Philadelphia (215) 243-2221
bet. 40th & 41st. in University City/W. Phila.

Votes are all over the map, at this "sometimes great, sometimes not" American/Italian, specializing in Pizza and a salad bar. While it does not win top marks for food, some call it their "favorite," especially for the newer, "gourmet"-style pizza toppings, like barbecue chicken. The room is below average, and the staff draws criticism, but they don't get in your way on the way to the salad bar that is "better than the pizza."

Bookbinder's Seafood House $34

215 S. 15th St., Philadelphia (215) 545-1137
at Walnut St. in Center City

"Good food and service," explains one voter of this Center City Continental Seafooder, but the "kitschy decor" needs a "facelift." A recent renovation did little to dispel these comments, yet it hasn't done anything to keep business lunchers, singles, and families with kids from frequenting owner Richard Bookbinder's "grand" room on 15th Street. Few surprises here, unless you count "disappointment;" you should reserve well in advance.

Boston Style Pizza $11

521 E. Lancaster Ave., Berwyn (610) 296-7082
across from Berwyn Shopping Ctr. on the Main Line

Ever wonder what pizza is like in Boston? Look no further than Nick Valavanis' Greek/Italian pizza spot in Berwyn. Within the plain walls of this little storefront, you'll find a "friendly" staff serving "good," consistent pizza day-in, day-out. We don't know what makes it "Boston-style," but we're guessing that "Berwyn-style" just doesn't sound as fancy.

FOOD ROOM STAFF COST

Brasil's

$25

112 Chestnut St., Philadelphia (215) 413-1700
at Front St. in the Historic Area

The food of Brazil is a prelude to the entertainment of Brazil at this Historic Area restaurant and night club, where you can "have a good meal and finish with a drink and dance upstairs," at least Wednesday through Saturday nights. The star of the menu is *feijoada,* the national dish, which combines greens and black beans with pork and sausage. Wash it down with *caipinha,* a close relative of the margarita, and finish with a *flan* before donning your dancing shoes.

Bravo Bistro

$26

175 King of Prussia Rd., Radnor Racquet Club, Radnor
(610) 293-9521
bet. Lancaster Ave. & Radnor-Chester Rd. on the Main Line

Some cry "Bravo for Bravo!" and say this Radnor Continental Bistro, which shares a kitchen with its formal sister, Passerelle, is a "fun, relaxing place to eat" "good, healthy meals." It has up to 20 wines by the glass and a "lovely location" overlooking a pond with swans. Even some who like the food say it's inconsistent and complain of "rude service" and "overcrowded" seating.

Brick Hotel

$31

Washington & State Sts., Newtown (215) 860-8313
in Bucks County

Set in a landmark-status historic structure, folks at the Brick Hotel have been serving good American food since 1764. While the menu isn't exactly revolutionary, this 13-room hotel is "a great getaway." After six years of new management, all reports indicate the quality is on a steady climb.

Bridget Foy's

$24

200 South St., Philadelphia (215) 922-1813
at 2nd St. in the South St. Area

The great people-watching at this South Street American is the major draw, though some voters claim that the "interesting selection" bears some "exceptional food," though the "whole menu is not great." That's a sign that this #10 restaurant for outdoor dining is bound for greatness, and that you should keep it simple or try the specials when ordering. Try it for Sunday brunch.

Bridgid's

$29

726 N. 24th St., Philadelphia (215) 232-3232
bet. Aspen & Fairmount in the Art Museum Area

This Art Museum area bistro is Philadelphia's only Belgian restaurant, meaning "the food is conceptually French, with portions to satisfy a German." What France is to wine, Belgium is to beer—many call it "the best beer selection in town." The bar food, among the survey's best, has a "constantly changing European flavor," and the $5 prix fixe lunch is "an amazing deal." Some call the casual room "only OK," but others say "wedding proposals are made at places like this." In this tiny place, reservations are a must.

= Superior = Excellent = Very Good

Brittingham's Irish Pub

$23

640 Germantown Pk., Lafayette Hill (610) 828-7351
in Montgomery County

If you're going to an Irish Pub, and expecting a four-star meal, then the problem is with you. If you're looking for "Guinness on tap and live Irish music," accompanied by "good burgers," a "good happy hour buffet" and even a "good Reuben," then you'll find none better than this Lafayette Hill spot. Oh, and if you can't get into the folk singers, belting out "great lush music," then go to the Fountain and shut up. P.S. St. Patty's Day is a mob scene.

Broad Axe Tavern

$21

Rt. 73 & Butler Pk., Broadaxe (215) 646-0477
in Montgomery County

While one voter says there's "nothing special here, just an extensive menu for picky families," most others agree it's a "good suburban local place," that's famous for its barbecue ribs and crabcakes. Well in the top 10 for barbecue, some go so far as to call it a "Montgomery County landmark," with "the best ribs anywhere." Jump off your diet, jump in the car, dress down, and head to Broadaxe.

Bruno's

$13

9800 Germantown Pk., Lafayette Hill (215) 242-1880
at Northeastern Ave. in Montgomery County

The brothers Bruno have created a "casual, relaxed" little Italian deli, that doubles in seating when the weather's nice. It's a "good family sandwich and salad place," and the view of Fairmount Park is the perfect complement to one of their hand-dipped ice cream cones.

Bubba's Pot Belly Stove

$21

1485 N. Rt. 309, Quakertown (215) 536-8308
in Bucks County

The stove isn't the only pot belly around this Quakertown Steak and Seafood joint: if what we hear about the "huge portions" is true, the patrons themselves run the risk of a bulging midriff. There is a certain kind of homeyness that you find only in a log cabin, which attracts the usual crowds of families at dinner but also interests the occasional businessperson at lunch.

Buck Hotel

$32

Bridgeton Rd.& Bustletown Pike, Feasterville (215) 322-5302
in Bucks County

While the food at this Feasterville American Continental might cost more than a buck, our voters commend the new management, particularly chef William Garber, for the "new and great" changes they have made. Wednesdays to Sundays, there's a jazz piano and vocalist, and all week they've got early bird specials, and kids are always welcome. P.S. the "catering service by Creative Cuisine is also excellent."

FOOD ROOM STAFF COST

Bunha Faun

$24

152 Lancaster Ave., Frazer (610) 651-2836
on the Main Line

Those who know about this small BYO French in Frazer aren't always inclined to tell. "We were tempted to keep it to ourselves," one ballot read, "but they deserve the recognition." Owner-chef Bungha Kuranaruk gives the cuisine Oriental overtones, and patrons appreciate the big portions and "comfortable decor." The place has drawbacks: a "limited menu" and a "smoky, dim" room, but most voters are surprised that "places with great food really exist all the way out there!"

Byrnes Tavern

$15

3301 Richmond St., Philadelphia (215) 634-8707
at Westmoreland St. in Port Richmond

Looks can be deceiving at this "dive"-cum-Top 10 crabhouse in Port Richmond. The American Tavern Fare, including (cleaned) crabs, wings and meats, is "very good," drawing a big crowd for a "congested eating area." P.S. This tavern is also known for its Irish Coffee.

Café Academie at the Doubletree Hotel

$23

Broad & Locust Sts., Philadelphia (215) 893-1667
in Center City

Voters are underwhelmed by the Contemporary American fare at this Center City hotel, and the room—the Doubletree Hotel's five-story atrium—gets only middling grades. But it stands across from the Academy of Music, so its curtain call menu comes in handy.

Café Arielle

$40

100 S. Main St., Doylestown (215) 345-5930
at Ashland St. in Bucks County

This "comfortable little place" in Doylestown's historic agricultural works building is Country French from its accordion music to its homemade pastries. The open kitchen specializes in grilled seafood and rotisserie poultry, and the menu also incorporates California touches to create "dishes you cannot cook at home."

Cafe Casa Nova

$19

1400 S. Delaware Ave., Phila. (215) 463-7707
at Reed St. in So. Phila.

Together, "Casanova" means "17th Century Italian Studboy." Separately, Casa Nova just means "new house." However, some people have the hots for this 3-year-old, Eurotech-looking regional Italian restaurant in South Philly. While the food gets consistently good ratings, not much stands out about the place, besides big portions and a decent wine by the glass selection.

= Superior = Excellent = Very Good

Cafe Einstein

$23

208 Race St., Philadelphia (215) 625-0904
at 2nd St. in the Historic Area

It doesn't take a genius to understand why this Old City Modern American has clicked with the "Philadelphia artsy" crowd who frequent the nearby galleries: the paintings on the exposed brick walls change monthly, the menu changes seasonally. Well-liked among older voters, for the wide selection of wines by the glass, and younger voters, who report that even "children have been there and like it."

Cafe Elana/Second Street Bistro

$26

414-16 S. 2nd St., Head House Sq., Philadelphia (215) 574-1687
bet. Pine & Lombard in the Historic Area

This Historic Area Italian has its fans, who praise the pasta, wish it were open for lunch and say the dining room overlooking Headhouse Square is "perfect for a romantic meal." But it also has an uncommon number of low scores, ("eh!", says one reviewer) indicating a problem with consistency.

Cafe Flower Shop

$18

2501 Meredith St., Philadelphia (215) 232-1076
bet. Fairmount & Aspen in the Art Museum Area

Dining among the blossoms at this Art Museum area homestyle American restaurant and working flower shop is like stepping into a Rousseau painting—there are "flowers and plants everywhere," so while you're sipping the wine you bring and the "wonderful homemade soups," you're also "given a lesson in basic botany." The most popular meal is Sunday brunch; regulars worry about the recent change in ownership, but those who've visited recently say "the new owners are great."

Café LaGrande

$21

240 Lancaster Ave., Malvern (610) 644-7333
at Rt. 401 on the Main Line

If you're looking for an inexpensive, buffet-style Continental restaurant in Malvern, then Café LaGrande (or, "the Big Cafe" to Francophobes) is for you. "Sunday brunch is a must for big appetites," but quantity over quality is "boring" to some of our voters.

Cafe Longano

$28

767 S. 9th St., Phila. (215) 440-9113 at Catherine St. in So. Phila.

While the food rating for this "homestyle" Abruzzi Italian may not be at the top of our lists, many of our voters think Longano's is "simply the best," though the "attentive staff" is usually the reason they give. You may recall that food is only part of "la dolce vita," and here, they focus on many of the other amenities, from a small but varied wine list, to good scotches and cognacs, and, of course, Sinatra on the sound system.

FOOD ROOM STAFF COST

Café Lutecia

$9

23rd & Lombard Sts., Philadelphia (215) 790-9557
in Center City

Chef/owner Valerie Blum has created a "friendly and comfortable" little neighborhood French spot on Lombard Street in Center City. It's a good pick for brunch, and the "unusual," "very good" sandwiches top many business lunchers' lists for top takeout. While they don't serve dinner, they're open all week for lunch and breakfast.

Cafe Michelangelo

$19

11901 Bustleton Ave., Philadelphia (215) 698-2233
Hendrix & Byberry in Northeast Phila.

While he was a damned good painter, Michelangelo was not known for his excellent cooking, and neither is this average, Regional Italian cafe in the Northeast. Still, it does some things very well, like the "very good" brick oven pizza that diners munch while watching Italian soccer on TV, or playing bocce ball out in the court.

Cafe 930

$9

930 Locust St., Philadelphia (215) 440-0930
bet. 9th & 10th in Center City

A low price tag for menu items complements the varied price tags on the frequently-changing artwork at this Mexican, Italian and American Cafe. Specializing in breakfast foods like muffins, croissants and pastries, and coffees from around the world, on the weekends they serve an especially good, relaxing breakfast ("no hurry, you have time to read the Sunday Inquirer"). Lunch served daily until 3:30.

Café Nola

$31

328 South St., Philadelphia (215) 627-2590
bet. 3rd & 4th in the South St. Area

Most Romac Reporters feel this mid-priced, very popular "Mardi Gras restaurant" does a very good job of bringing "authentic New Orleans cuisine" to South Street. Even those who think the servers "act as if they're doing you a favor" give high marks for the food, especially the soft-shell crabs. While some think the room is "romantic," others find it "cramped" and "a bit noisy." For most, a visit is "the next best thing to being on Bourbon Street." One of the area's top three brunch restaurants.

Cafe on Quince

$22

202 S. Quince St., Philadelphia (215) 592-1750
Walnut & 11th & 12th in Center City

Just like the theaters in the area around this Eclectic American, they're closed on Mondays. And, just like the theaters, the substance of the fare takes a back seat to the show: the staff easily wins out over the food and room. "Worth the trip down a dark alley," say our voters, appreciating the reasonable prices and the many low-cost specials—when else—pre-theater.

Cafe Piazza

$21

2227 Pine St., Philadelphia (215) 546-2547
at 23rd St. in Center City

Romac Reporters call this casual but romantic Italian in Southwest Center City with a view of the fountain in Fitler Square a "nice neighborhood restaurant" with a "good bar" and a nice selection of wines by the glass. A few think it's overpriced, but others say it's a "great value," especially at Saturday and Sunday brunch.

Cafe Preeya

$25

2651 Huntingdon Pk., Village Center Shopping Ctr., Huntingdon Valley (215) 947-6195
Above Red Lion Rd. in Montgomery County

With good food ratings, especially from diners under 30, chef/owner Preeya Chanyothi has put together an "outstanding find" in Huntington Valley. The "innovative menu" contains items like buffalo, in addition to a wide fish selection. Older voters think the place could use a sprucing up, but all agree that the food is "consistently good," with great selections from the Jefferson Heart Menu. Bring your own, but not on Monday when it's closed.

Cafe San Pietro

VOTE

41 W. Lancaster Ave., across from the movie theater, Ardmore (610) 896-4740 (on the Main Line)

While this Southern Italian restaurant in Ardmore is too new to have made our poll, we've heard great things by word of mouth. With little granite tables and an oak bar, this small trattoria serves hot and cold sandwiches, salads, pastas, and in the evenings, chicken, fish and veal. Their reasonable prices have made this place popular, and they have plans to expand in 1996.

Cafe Sorella

$20

314 N. 4th St., Philadelphia (215) 592-7075
at Wood St. in the Historic Area

With few fans and consistent, if only fair ratings, we wonder what keeps Sorella going. According to our reviewers, they have recently revamped the menu, keeping the favorites and moving toward an less-expensive, lighter board. Still finding its feet, the sisters may yet be to your liking.

Cafette

$14

8136 Ardleigh St., Philadelphia (215) 242-4220
Hartwell Ln. & Abington in Chestnut Hill/Mt. Airy
2816 DeKalb Pk., East Norriton (610) 277-9948
in Montgomery County
Shurs Lane & Terrace St., Phila. (215) 487-9572
in Manayunk/Roxborough

The scores are all over the map for these eclectic cafes, with "highly variable food—sometimes great," sometimes not. The menu, which lists homemade favorites from fried chicken to vegetable lasagna, and "very relaxed atmosphere" make it "great for young families," even if they're not crazy about the "homey" but "cramped" dining rooms.

FOOD ROOM STAFF COST

Cafe Zesty
$25

4382 Main St., Philadelphia (215) 483-6226 in Manayunk

Once again, Romac Reporters wrestled with the Greco-Roman cuisine at this Manayunk spot, and the results were again a draw. Voters like the seafood, "perfect" bread, Greek salads and wines; to others the food is "bland, bland, bland." The restaurant used to be crowded but recently doubled in size; that might help improve service scores.

Caffe Raffaelo
$20

8080 Old York Rd., Elkins Pk (215) 782-1950 in Montgomery Co.

What can you say about an mid-sized, mid-priced Italian in Northeast Philly? That it has prix fixe menu specials, kids specials, and easy listening on the stereo? Nothing special there. If you figure it out, tell us.

Canal House
$24

30 W. Mechanic St., New Hope (215) 862-2069 at New St. in Bucks Co.

This Northern Italian, with an Eclectic (though primarily Continental) flair is a prime spot for outdoor dining on the canal. Closing in on its fiftieth year, it's a lovely stop in the wintertime, too, with two "cozy fireplaces," and a lovely, country setting.

Capital Vietnam
$14

1008 Race St., Phila. (215) 925-2477 bet. 10th & 11th in Chinatown

The decor won't turn any heads at this Chinatown Vietnamese; go for "good, cheap Asian eats." Voters say it's a good spot for those learning the ins and outs of Vietnamese cuisine—"the waiters will guide you" on what to order and how to eat it.

Capriccio
$11

17th & Locust, Warwick Hotel, Phila. (215) 735-9797 in Ctr. City

The ratings aren't bad for a coffee shop, but voters expect more from a place with such a prime location. "They fire their staff regularly," says one, and that's a good comment. Though you might never spend more than $10 here, voters still think it's "waaay expensive."

Caribou Café
$17

1126 Walnut St., Phila. (215) 625-9535 (bet. 11th & 12th in Ctr. City)

"All that's missing is Kerouac" from this "cool and hip" French Bistro in Center City. With French, jazz or classical music on the sound system, this "very Euro" spot offers "chic yet tasty" food in a "good Nouveau atmosphere," at a low price that's a "great bang for the buck." It's a "favorite Center City rendezvous."

Carlino's Specialty Foods
$17

2612 E. County Ln. Rd., Ardmore (610) 649-4046
bet. Ardmore & Haverford Aves. on the Main Line

This Main Line takeout shop is "the best Italian takeout and deli" around, "great for when you don't want to cook." It's also extremely popular, so if you "avoid the Saturday afternoon zoo," you might join the chorus that sings, "Carlino's is heaven!"

 = Superior = Excellent = Very Good

Carolina's

$26

261 S. 20th St., Philadelphia (215) 545-1000
bet. Locust & Spruce Sts. in Center City
Something could be finer than the only-average ratings across the board for this much-trafficked though small "refined homestyle" American. It's in our Top 10 for both conversation and singles pickups, though one voter notes it may be "stuck in the '80s." Though "crowded," and "a bit pretentious for my comfort zone," many diners seem to find some satisfaction from this "neighborhood hangout."

Carolina's

$28

333 Belrose Ln., Radnor (610) 293-1000
at King of Prussia Rd. on the Main Line
The Radnor branch of this Regional American scores about the same as its Center City sibling. Though "they do grilled food well" and the "veal loaf is great," many complain of "small portions" and say the food is "too precious" and sometimes arrives cold because of inconsistent service.

Carversville Inn

$33

Carversville & Aquetong Rds., Carversville (215) 297-0900
in Bucks County
It wasn't easy finding reviewers for this small (seats 50) restaurant located so far out of town. Those who voted agree that the Regional American (mainly Southern) dishes, were very good. Staff also receives high marks. Lovely, historic, and open every day but Monday.

Cary

$25

211 S. 15th St., Phila. (215) 735-9100
Walnut & Locust in Center City
This new Center City New World/Pacific Rim Grill is upscale, but with enough casual touches to make it comfortable and fun. The room is lovely, with flowers and linen tablecloths, connected to an open kitchen that provides an "interesting, informal atmosphere," including floor-to-ceiling windows. There's also sidewalk dining in the good weather. "Excellent presentation" starts with a "very good" staff, and they even have cigar dinners, like stuffier spots in the area.

Casa Mexicana

$20

111 Cotton St., Philadelphia (215) 487-1009
Crescent & Main in Manayunk/Roxborough
Coming up on ten years in business, this Manayunk Mexican pulls in big crowds, though it's not for any of the usual criteria our participants vote on. The food is only "fair," the atmosphere a bit "creepy," and the staff is below average. Portions are called "minimal," and it's "expensive for Mexican," compared with others in the area. Live bands, margaritas and a late closing time are the draws here.

= Good **= Fair** **[no rating] = Poor**

FOOD ROOM STAFF COST

Cascade Lodge

$40

5065 Lehnenberg Rd., Kintnersville (610) 346-7484
at Rt. 611 in Bucks County

This Continental in the wilds of Bucks County features "great food," views of the "beautiful grounds" and the freshest trout you'll find anywhere—you net your own from a spring that runs through the wine cellar. The best cooking is tableside; the experience is "superb and fun," "very romantic" and "worth the ride." Jacket required.

Casey's Dugout

$17

516 King St., Paoli (610) 644-3084 (on the Main Line)

Our reviewers gave Mighty Casey another swing at the ball, and it's a hit, if only an infield grounder. Follow your instincts at this all-baseball themed restaurant, and stick with burgers, steaks, and the "best crabcakes," that really do win waves of raves.

Casey's Rest. & Saloon

$19

812 Lansdowne Ave., Drexel Hill (610) 789-7575
at State Rd. in Delaware County

This casual Drexel Hill American pulls in customers with "good prime rib, reasonably priced." The kids' menu makes it a good family spot early in the evening; a DJ provides entertainment Thursday through Saturday.

Cassatt Tea Room

$23

210 W. Rittenhouse Sq., The Rittenhouse, Philadelphia
(215) 546-9000 in Center City

In the mood for tiny, open-faced sandwiches? This "elegant and quiet tea room" is the next best thing to being in England, without the onerous taxes, nationalized health and the tabloid press. You can even have tea outside in the garden in nice weather. With miniature pastries, finger sandwiches, scones and preserves, if you want a "quiet, relaxing and undiscovered tea room," this is the real thing.

Casselli's

$26

7620 Ridge Ave., Phila. (215) 483-6969 (in Manayunk/Roxborough)

This Roxborough Italian is "often crowded" because, while it doesn't take reservations, it has plenty of fans who think its "atmosphere is a gas," resulting in "long waits on weekends." "Huge portions" of "homemade Italian" dishes get high marks, but people go home talking about the singer—some think it's "fantastic" and "entertaining," others say it's "too loud" and "cheesy." All agree the place is run by "nice people" who "make you feel at home."

Catalina, The Grill at

$24

2001 Hamilton St., Korman Suites Hotel, Philadelphia
(215) 569-7500 (at 20th St. in the Art Museum Area)

Well it IS a grill... but it's actually near the Art Museum, and finds itself in the tourist category for that area. Few people consider this place any more than average, and it has plenty of detractors. A recent renovation puts the "shabby" room rating in doubt.

 = Superior = Excellent = Very Good

Catfish Cafe & Steakhouse

$28

4007 Ridge Ave., Philadelphia (215) 229-9999
at Scotts Ln. in East Falls

The century-old mahogany bar sets the tone for "a good funky-atmosphere place" at this Eclectic American in East Falls. Such an "out-of-the-way location" is a hindrance for some, but others swear it's "worth the trip to sample the blackened catfish." Steak is another favorite. For an inexpensive taste, try the prix fixe menu in the bar on weeknights.

Cavanaugh's

$13

119 S. 39th St., Philadelphia (215) 386-4889
39th & Sansom Sts. in University City/W. Phila.

Simple pleasures are the best, especially when it comes to the burgers, pastas and seafood at this University City American. While it doesn't pull down good ratings, it is not without its good points, like "the best coconut shrimp" and a "huge beer selection" at the "great bar."

Cedar's

$17

616 S. 2nd St., Philadelphia (215) 925-4950
bet. South & Bainbridge Sts. in the South St. Area

"Friendly, reliable, delicious and inexpensive... what more could you ask for?" inquires one reviewer, who has obviously turned a blind eye to the crummy decor and so-so service. So what has preserved Cedar's for the last ten years on South Street? Great "spinach pies and homemade hummus," at a "great value." One voter advises you "order everything—they have the best *taboulleh* anywhere!"

Celebre's Pizzeria

$12

1536 Packer Ave., Packer Park Shopping Ctr., Philadelphia (215) 467-3255 15th & Packer in So. Phila.

Owner Robert Celebre has made this joint a part of the Philadelphia experience, and he's done it all with very good pizza. Simply put, he has the "best pizza and the best people," especially before or after a game at the Spectrum or the Vet. Stop by and check out his numerous awards—that's about all there is for decor.

Cent'Anni

$27

770 S. 7th St., Philadelphia (215) 925-5558
bet. Fitzwater & Catherine in So. Phila.

The young owners of this South Philly Italian have breathed some California influences and fresh herbs into the "trattoria cuisine," and reviewers say that watching the food being prepared makes them feel like they're "sitting in an Italian kitchen." Voters are split on the exposed-brick, tin-ceilinged room: What's "cozy dining" for some is "a little tight" for others. Prices aren't bad, and there are toys and coloring books to keep kids busy.

FOOD ROOM STAFF COST

Central Bar & Grille

$25

39 Morris Ave., Bryn Mawr (610) 527-1400
Across from Bryn Mawr Train Station on the Main Line

Centrally located in Bryn Mawr, this Contemporary American has some diehard fans, whose top ratings are pulled down by an equal number of dissenters in the huge group of voters. The same owner as Bravo Bistro/Passerelle has packed a lot of features into this 1890s freighthouse baggage building: with kid-friendly, "off-the-wall" train decor, good microbrew and wine by the glass selection, and much more, diners advise Central to "simplify."

Century House

VOTE

Rt. 309, Hatfield (215) 822-0139
in Montgomery County

This Montco American hangs its hat on its bargain early bird specials, offered every night plus all day Sunday. A dozen choices at $13.95 range from standards like steak au poivre to trendier dishes like grilled pork with sweet potato fries. Voters say the very good food and "quiet atmosphere" attract a "mostly older clientele."

Chadds Ford Inn

$31

Rts 1 & 100 , Chadds Ford (610) 388-7361
in Delaware County

This historic inn in Chester County's Wyeth country serves "outstanding" Continental and regional food with a fresh, light touch in "simple surroundings" that "feel like a real country inn." The tavern has a cheaper, more casual menu; it's also the only place where you can smoke. The crossroads complex includes an art gallery and shops for browsing, or "you can linger in the bar over a great cup of one of their specialty coffees."

Chadds Ford Tavern

$26

RD 2 Box 96A, Chadds Ford (610) 459-8453
Baltimore Pk. & Harvey Rd. in Delaware County

There are two sides to the food at the Chadds Ford Tavern. The first is the "good sandwiches" and other pub food in the bar, which is also the home to much of the place's history. In the dining room, you'll find decent Continental food, "really good," they say, but with "not much ambiance." Two charcoal pits and bread baked on premises give the place a homey feel.

Chambers

$22

19 N. Main St., Doylestown (215) 348-1940
at State St. in Bucks County

Eclectic elements go into making what's good at this little Doylestown restaurant. It's everything we've come to expect from a spot that specializes in catering: a casual feel (with light jazz on the stereo), good Sunday brunches, reasonable wines and special, homemade desserts. Bring the kids, and if they let you (the kids, that is), relax.

Chancery

$23

15 S. High St., West Chester (610) 344-0530
at Market St. in Chester County

With chef changes in the works, the food rating gets tossed out, but, based on the other elements, this big West Chester Continental/American is worth a visit. Ratings and comments agree, the renovated historic building provides "great atmosphere," along with the Earl Rice Quintet on Friday nights. With a great baked brie appetizer, we have a feeling Chancery's about to lose the title of "the best-kept secret in West Chester."

Chanterelles

$50

1312 Spruce St., Philadelphia (215) 735-7551
bet. 13th & Broad in Center City

Named for the tasty French mushroom, the site of this teensy Center City French gave Le Bec Fin and La Panatiere their starts, and indeed, some think chef Philippe Chin has improved upon those originals. But remember, dear reader, for "presentation that is second to none," of "nearly perfect food and service," don't forget to "bring your credit card" to this "romantic" and very special place. Hey, if you're on a mileage program, dinner for two will get you halfway to France.

Charles Plaza

$17

236 N. 10th St., Philadelphia (215) 829-4383
at Vine St. in Chinatown

This Chinatown spot stands out because the menu is about 75 percent vegetarian, creating "a more relaxed brown rice Chinese" than some all-vegetarian spots nearby. Healthy cooking is emphasized even on the meat dishes ("try the chicken with ginger and pear"). Food is "light and very fresh," prepared with sea salt and raw brown sugar and without fat or MSG. Plus "knowledgeable and friendly" owner Charles Chen makes a "charming host."

Charlotte's

$23

3207 W. Chester Pk., Newtown Square (610) 356-7100
in Delaware County

While the price may be low for a Continental restaurant (with French touches) in Newtown Square, the ratings are consistently below-average. Though the experience may be "pleasant," with a "varied menu," there are no surprises, and most of our voters seem to think the "mediocre" food and atmosphere "need to be updated." You must reserve, and for a cheap look at the place, you might try the early bird specials.

Chart House

$35

555 South Columbus Blvd., Philadelphia (215) 625-8383
at Penn's Landing on the Delaware Riverfront

This Penn's Landing Steak and Seafood spot impresses voters with "the sweetest view in town"—it was No. 1 in the survey. But many say that, with the exception of the salad bar (also No. 1), "the view outshines the food," which is "routine" and "overpriced." Some avoid the problem by coming for Sunday brunch or just coffee and dessert, especially the mud pie.

FOOD ROOM STAFF COST

Chef Charin

$22

126 Bala Ave., Bala Cynwyd (610) 667-8680
bet. Montgomery & City Line Aves. on the Main Line

This new Bala Cynwyd spot offers a Continental menu, but the most popular items are unique fusions of Thai and Italian influences, such as Ping Pong Pasta, pasta with seafood in a creamy Thai-seasoned sauce. Though some think the kitchen is trying to do too much, most find "this is a pleasant surprise; the food is fresh, tasty and interesting." "Nice—and BYOB keeps costs down."

Chef's Market

$15

231 South St., Philadelphia (215) 925-8360
bet. 2nd & 3rd. Sts. in the South St. Area

South Street's upscale food market is heat 'n' eat nirvana—60 to 80 different items, ranging from entrees and side dishes to appetizers and dessert, so you can assemble an entire dinner party, right down to the cheese course. It's also "nice to eat *al fresco*" (at a table on the sidewalk)—"too bad it's dirty South Street." Our voters say it's a little pricey, but they "love it for the great selection."

Chef Tell's Harrow Inne

$48

Rts. 611 & 412, Ottsville (610) 847-2464
in Bucks County

Tell Erhardt's country inn in Ottsville is a "quaint, artsy building," but the eclectic menu combines everything from Pacific Rim and Cajun dishes to "unique German fare." The result, voters say, is "enjoyable" and "memorable" if a little "inconsistent," and it's "a good place to go if you want to meet a celebrity chef."

Cherry Street Chinese Vegetarian

$16

1010 Cherry St., Philadelphia (215) 923-3663
bet. 10th & 11th in Chinatown

Number Five for Vegetarian food in our City-wide poll, this meatless Chinese is referred to by our voters as "the best Vegetarian Chinese." In fact, one reviewer goes as far as to say it is "without a doubt, the best choice for vegetarians and kosher persons!" Meat-lovers will be pleasantly surprised by the wonderfully flavorful (and healthy) food, and penny-pinchers will love the inexpensive bill, and the BYOB policy.

Chesapeake Bay Seafood Hse.

$22

735 Middletown Blvd., Langhorne (215) 752-2005
at Rt. 1 in Bucks County

Woof! Looking over the numbers, it's hard to believe that anybody would have any nice comments about this Langhorne Seafood spot, but we hear it's "good for what it is: a family seafood restaurant with unlimited seconds." "Take the kids here," and bring along your Homer Simpson-sized appetite: If you make a scene you don't have to worry about never coming back.

Chili's

$16

38th & Chestnut, Phila. (215) 222-7322 (in U. City/W. Phila.)
739 W. DeKalb Pk., K. of Prussia (610) 992-0899 (in Mont. Co.)
312 Lancaster Ave., Wayne (610) 687-1001 (on the Main Line)
175 City Ave., Bala Cynwyd (610) 667-4444 (in the City Line Area)

Chili's scores look unimpressive until they're stacked up against similar chains' scores. While some voters have "awful" experiences, many say it's "a great place to take the kids—$1 per!" The food isn't great, but it's "better than you'd expect," and "children and parents can both enjoy it and be comfortable."

Chris' Jazz Cafe

$22

1421 Sansom St., Philadelphia (215) 568-3131 in Center City

"Jazz" comes before "cafe" here for good reason. This Center City bar/restaurant has "great music," Tuesday through Saturday nights and even at lunch, Monday through Thursday, with the "great host," Chris, running the show. However, the American food with Oriental flair is mostly ignored by the jazz-loving patrons.

Chubby's Steaks

$11

5826 Henry Ave., Philadelphia (215) 487-2575
at Walnut Ln. in Manayunk/Roxborough

Voters are cool to the formica-and-tile decor at this Roxborough cheesesteak and hoagie joint, but they love that it's open 'til the wee hours, calling it a "cool late-night, after-bar place." Unlike most hoagie shops, it offers a wide variety of beers, both bottled and on tap.

Chumley's at the Sheraton Valley Forge

$31

1116 N. First Ave., King of Prussia (610) 337-2000
at N. Gulph Rd. in Montgomery County

This Steak and Seafooder in the Valley Forge Sheraton pulls in the locals with classy decor—mahogany-paneled walls, etched glass, chandeliers. The food scores are more ho-hum, but some say Chumley's offers a "good quantity of food at reasonable prices."

Chun Hing

$16

4160 Monument Rd., Pathmark Supercenter, Philadelphia
(215) 879-6270 (beh. the Adams Mark Hotel in City Line Area)

Owner Tony Hong is also the chef at this casual City Line area Chinese, which specializes in spicy Szechuan cuisine (though they'll make dishes mild at your request). Many say it's the "best Chinese in the area" and the "staff is sweet," a few say the kitchen is "inconsistent."

Churrasqueira Vila Verde

VOTE

1211 S. Bethlehem Pk., Ambler (215) 643-3661
at Butler Pk. in Montgomery County

This Portuguese recently relocated to a spot in Ambler with an indoor pit grill so it could cook in traditional Portuguese style. Voters say the food is "flavorful" and "authentic, especially the seafood dishes," but most also say it's "a bit pricey" for a BYOB.

= Good **= Fair** **[no rating] = Poor**

FOOD ROOM STAFF COST

Ciboulette

$49

200 S. Broad St., The Bellevue, Philadelphia (215) 790-1210
at Walnut St. in Center City

"Subtle, sublime" French Provincial food with an Asian accent served in Center City's historic Bellevue Hotel makes Ciboulette one of the best in the book. A five-course prix fixe menu is offered at $60, plus a wine list with "great bargains," are for those who want to experience "perfection on a plate" without spending a fortune. The original tile floor, while beautiful, does make the room noisy, but "superlative service" has voters crying out, "Give Bruce Lim a fifth star!"

Circa

$32

1518 Walnut St., Phil. (215) 545-6800 (bet. 15th & 16th in Ctr. City)

Circa receives good marks for its food, but the real story is the ambiance: It's an after-work/nighttime singles mecca. With a bar that was "designed for a church," Circa's many fans recommend you "ask to eat in the vault," or try the "great people-watching in the club upstairs." You don't have to be young and single to enjoy the creative American food, however, and business diners like it for lunch.

City Tavern

$31

138 S. 2nd St., Philadelphia (215) 413-1443
at Walnut St. in the Historic Area

This Colonial-era tavern would be included on tours of the Historic Area even if it were empty—after all, the Founding Fathers actually supped and sipped within these walls. Every room has a fireplace, servers wear Colonial garb and harpsichord music fills the air Friday and Saturday nights. The menu is just as authentic, but it's not stiff or stodgy—"the lobster pie is to die for," the "pepper pot soup is outstanding" and a kids' menu makes it suitable for families. It all adds up to an "interesting place to take out-of-towners," or anyone looking for a brush, and a bite, with history.

Classic Diner, The

VOTE

352 Lancaster Ave., Malvern (610) 725-0515 (on the Main Line)

This throwback to the old roadhouse/diner is too new to rate. It's a small cottage on Rt. 30, with an old-fashioned soda fountain, eggs for breakfast, and all the other comfort food you'd expect. The modern twist—brick oven pizza. Let us know what you think on your questionnaire next year.

Clemente's

$32

116 E. Gay St., West Chester (610) 344-7644
bet. Matlack & Walnut Sts. in Chester County

Check out the gold records for owner Bill Blough (of George Thorogood's band): many of our voters feel this place deserves them for the food, rooms and staff. Set in an historic building, the Northern Italian/Continental menu pulls down big ratings, especially when you consider the moderate price tag. One diner calls it "the best food to value ratio," and though it's "intimate and romantic," there's also a place for pipe and cigar smokers.

 = Superior = Excellent = Very Good

Cock 'n Bull

$29

Rt. 202 & Street Rd., Peddlar's Village, Lahaska (215) 794-4010 in Bucks County

Peddler Village's lower-priced, Country American has a reputation as "the place to take your parents on a Sunday afternoon," but it actually scores slightly higher among younger voters. The menu features "classic American dining choices" like chicken pot pie and cinnamon bread, cooked at an open hearth that adds ambiance. Some scoff that it "caters to tourists," only natural given its location in a Central Bucks attraction that features specialty shops, an antique carousel and a carousel museum.

Colombia Hotel

$32

148 Bridge St., Phoenixville (610) 933-9973 at Rt. 29 in Chester County

Unlike many historic buildings, this American Steak and Seafood spot in Phoenixville hasn't had a recent renovation. Some reviewers like the "old-time Victorian elegance," especially the bar's old-world charm; others think it's getting "shabby." There's no disagreement over the "modern, delicious meals"—it's "all-American food with a creative twist" and some of the "best seafood in the 'burbs."

Concordville Inn

$32

Rts. 1 & 322, Concordville (610) 459-2230 in Delaware County

"Good food and good prices," plus the ability to seat 2,000 people, have made this huge American/Continental country inn a popular choice in Concordville. The private rooms appeal to the corporate meeting planners, the 200-plus-year-old structure, with an adjoining 117 room English Inn, appeals to the history buffs, and the $13.95 family night specials appeal to just about everybody else.

Conti Cross Keys Inn

$36

Rts. 611 & 313, Doylestown (215) 348-9600 in Bucks County

The crossed keys—a symbol of hospitality, as on a concierge's collar—is appropriate to this welcoming Continental American in Doylestown. They actually take the name from the Coat of Arms of the papal see, and some folks have downright religious experiences with the "very good" food. With a very good staff, there are few surprises, except that for some, the "prices are high."

Continental Restaurant & Martini Bar

VOTE

2nd & Market Sts., Philadelphia (215) 923-6069 in the Historic Area

Too new for our survey, this swank martini-themed International is housed in an old stainless steel diner, but is tricked-out in style. There are a couple hundred martini glasses hanging over the old lunch counter, the lights over the booths are olives stuck with giant toothpicks, and the olive booths have pimento pinstripes. The kitchen serves "world plates"—small tapas portions, for patrons to mix and match. Open 'til 1:00 a.m. for late snacks, Mon.-Sat, and until an ultra-civilized 4:00 p.m. for Sunday brunch.

= Good = Fair [no rating] = Poor

FOOD ROOM STAFF COST

Copabanana/ Copa Pronto

$15

4th & South Sts., Phila. (215) 923-6180 in the South St. Area

Though the signature Margaritas are "lethal," plenty of our voters, particularly the young ones, have survived long enough to go back time and again to this South Street Tex-Mex/burger joint. In our Top 10 for Best Bar Food and Best Dive, this "dark, smoke filled" place is characterized by "bad service," and one sedate partyer recommends that you "visit on a weekday for a more tolerable atmosphere."

Copa, Too!

$15

263 S. 15th St., Phila. (215) 735-0848
bet. Locust & Spruce in Center City

This Center City Tex/Mex bar rates only fair for food, service and ambiance. So what's the attraction? "Order up the margaritas—they're the finest" in what others call Center City's "premier beer bar." Voters are lukewarm on the "slightly jazzed-up pub grub"; they suggest that you stick to the burgers, Spanish fries and hot wings.

Coppermill Harvest at the Park Ridge

VOTE

480 N. Gulph Rd., King of Prussia (610) 337-1800
at Rt. 202 in Montgomery County

This King of Prussia American reels in customers with buffets: "A seafood lover's delight on Saturday night," Italian on Friday night and an "exceptional" brunch on Sunday. The lounge is a bar with shuffleboard, electronic darts and pool tables.

Country Club Rest. & Pastry Shop

$15

1717 Cottman Ave., Philadelphia (215) 722-0500
at Summerdale St. in Northeast Phila.

Celebrating 40 years as the Northeast's only Jewish-American diner, this Cottman Avenue landmark is open 7:00 a.m. 'til 1:00 a.m., 7 days. You "get your money's worth," from "great breakfasts" to "kasha and bow ties." While the food rates just "fair," all the talk is about the "fresh desserts," that might include the "best cheesecake in town."

Country House Inn

$31

1330 W. Baltimore Pk., Wawa (610) 358-1138 (in Delaware Cty.)

This rambling Victorian Wawa steak and seafood spot earns just average scores, but it has something for everyone—a fixed-price dinner, a kids' menu, and a variety of dining environments, including a greenhouse room and a Tiffany room featuring tiffany lamps. And it does all this at mid-level prices.

Country Squire Diner

$15

Rts. 3 & 320, Broomall (610) 353-0550 (in Delaware County)

Just like the station wagon of the same name, this Top 10 Romac diner in Broomall is a popular family choice. From "delicious grilled chicken Caesar salad" to "great Napoleons" and other desserts, this place "has everything" in diner food. A few naysayers voted low, bringing the ratings down a bit. Open 24/7, try the "breakfast at 11pm."

 = Superior = Excellent = Very Good

Courtyard Cafe

$27

1 Logan Sq., Philadelphia (215) 963-1500 (in Center City)
What distinguishes the Courtyard Cafe from any other light lunch spot? Just that it's an outdoor cafe, that it serves "Chef's picnic fare" from one of the best kitchens in the country, and that it's the highest rated lunch spot on the survey. Open May through September.

Coventry Forge Inn

$45

3360 Coventryville Rd., Pottstown (610) 469-6222
N. of Rt. 23 in Montgomery County
Pottstown's premier French restaurant has just passed the forty year mark and is still going strong. "Worth the drive" is only the beginning of the praise that Romac Reporters lavish on this "elegant, quiet, romantic" spot. They also love the very old setting, calling it "the place that started it all" and "one of my all-time favorites." The "unique, natural setting" also includes rooms for a cozy overnight.

Crier in the Country

$37

Rt. 1, Baltimore Pk., Glen Mills (610) 358-2411
bet. Rts. 261 & 322 in Delaware County
The historic Delaware County building cries out "upscale understated elegance," but a recent switch to Continental and Regional American fare still leaves voters saying "too expensive for the quality of food." The "gorgeous" setting gets higher marks, one reason the Crier is popular for parties and weddings.

Cuisines

$29

200 Wilmington-W. Chester Pk., Chadds Ford (610) 459-3397
Rts. 202 & 491 in Delaware County
The "attentive staff" and "delicate decor" get good grades, but a wide-ranging international menu—"almost too much to select from"—is the lure at this Chadds Ford Contemporary. But while voters rave about the "clever cuisine," they're split on the live jazz on weekends.

Cutillo's

$26

2688 E. High St., Pottstown (610) 327-2910
at Sanatoga Rd. in Montgomery County
You may not have gone to heaven, but you will hear harp music on Friday and Saturday nights at this Pottstown neighborhood American. Set in a wooded area with a stream running through, it features a "good selection, and good servers," too. Comfortable and tucked away, you feel special here even if the food does not.

Cuttalossa Inn

$39

River Rd., Lumberville (215) 297-5082
Six miles N. of New Hope in Bucks County
The nearly-$40 price tag for the no better than average American cuisine at this large, Bucks County restaurant in an 1820's building has our viewers screaming "overpriced." Actually, they just yell that—they scream "it's hard to believe the prices for this food." Cut your losses.

= Good = Fair [no rating] = Poor

FOOD ROOM STAFF COST

Cutter's

$28

2005 Market St., One Commerce Sq., Philadelphia (215) 851-6262
at 20th St. in Center City

Romac Reporters rank Cutter's "spectacular bar" the No. 1 singles bar in the area ("an executive spawning pond," one sniffed), as well as the best place for an after-work drink, but it's also a good spot for business meals because the food is more than an afterthought. Much of it is cooked over a wood-fired grill; voters rave about the "best salmon in Philly" and say "gorgonzola potatoes are a treat." The only negative reviews come from those who think it's "too glitzy."

Dahlak

$14

4708 Baltimore Ave., Philadelphia (215) 726-6464
Cedar & Springfield Sts. in University City/W. Phila.

This Ethiopian is in a dicey area, but voters say "don't let the neighborhood daunt you." The "consistently wonderful" exotic fare and "always friendly" service make for an evening that's "adventurous and worth it," especially at such rock-bottom prices.

Dalessandro's Steaks

$8

600 Wendover St., Philadelphia (215) 482-5407
Henry Ave. & Walnut Ln. in Manayunk/Roxborough

A top 5 contender for best cheesesteak in Philly (and clearly the best steaks in Roxborough), this Cheesesteak and Hoagie joint is "always packed," and though they may have the "best pepper selection," it is the cheesesteaks that keep 'em waddling back for more. "Best steak sandwiches" is repeated by our voters like a mantra, though they get creative with the expletives when it comes to the room and the staff.

D'Angelo's

$30

256 S. 20th St., Philadelphia (215) 546-3935
bet. Spruce & Locust Sts. in Center City

This Center City Italian, where the owner likes to bring out his guitar after 10 p.m., strikes a chord with some voters—"some of the finest Italian food and ambiance anywhere," "as good as there is, especially if you like appetizers." Naysayers pull the ratings down to just "good." The service earns decent scores, but some feel the long, narrow rooms "leave a lot to be desired."

D'Angelo's Summit

$19

8100 Ridge Ave., Philadelphia (215) 482-5323
at Summit Ave. in Manayunk/Roxborough

Low prices don't seem to make up for low ratings at this Roxborough American/Continental/Italian, according to most of our voters. Still, it's a "good neighborhood restaurant" with "many choices," starting with the "great salad and soup bar" and graduating up to the "homestyle" if "blah" Italian cooking. This summit is fraught with many valleys.

= Superior = Excellent = Very Good

Dante and Luigi's

$22

762 S. 10th St., Philadelphia (215) 922-9501
at Catharine St. in So. Phila.

Some regulars have been eating at this South Philly Italian since they were tots for "fabulous Italian food at a cook-it-yourself price." Others say the food is "inconsistent," but is offset by "great waiters" and "quiet atmosphere." Sinatra-era music adds to the nostalgic atmosphere.

Dardanelles

$18

213 Chestnut St., Philadelphia (215) 925-8333
at Strawberry St. in the Historic Area

This Society Hill BYO is called "the Turkish counterpart to Dmitri's" for its smallish room and spectacular grilled fish, especially octopus, that's "inexpensive and delicious, homestyle and lots of fun!" The husband-and-wife team of Levent and Sherri Yueksel keep out the crowds by refusing to advertise—there isn't even a sign out front!

Dave & Buster's

$20

325 N. Columbus Blvd., Pier 19 N., Philadelphia (215) 413-1951
bet. Race & Spring Garden Sts. on the Delaware Riverfront

"An overpriced place for overgrown kids (i.e. grownups)," writes one diner, "but still fun." Keep it simple both with the food and the wide array of entertainment, from virtual reality games to a no-money casino, and watch it—"this place can get expensive." Name it and they've got it, from Karaoke to Murder Mystery nights—though some say it can be "a dumb show." Nonetheless, this "Chuck E. Cheese for adults" is in the top 10 for bar food, and is number 1 for children.

Day by Day

$14

21st & Sansom Sts., Philadelphia (215) 564-5540
in Center City

Oh, dear lord, we pray that people understand the ratings at this very, very Nouvelle Eclectic restaurant in Center City. With a menu that changes, well, day by day, you will find few old time favorites here, but you can count on "great lunches," and quiche after quiche after quiche.

Dean & DeLuca

$12

251 S. 18th St., Philadelphia Art Alliance Bldg., Philadelphia (215) 893-1420 (bet. Spruce & Locust Sts. in Center City)
1601 Market St., Phila. (215) 563-7755 (at 16th St. in Center City)
4311 Main St., Phila. (215) 487-2078 (in Manayunk/Roxborough)

The light fare at these Center City gourmet food emporia receives good marks; many say the 18th street branch, the dining room of a turn-of-the-century mansion, makes it "a lovely place for a party and an unknown gem for lunch." But the top draw here is the coffee—#1 for espresso/cappuccino, and the #1 coffeehouse on our survey. However, some complain "portions are too small," it's "overpriced," and "the food is much better in the New York store." Voters chide the staff—"service is slow," "needs attitude adjustment."

= Good = Fair [no rating] = Poor

FOOD ROOM STAFF COST

Deetrick's

VOTE

211 Old York Rd., Jenkintown (215) 576-7690
in Montgomery County

This new jazz cafe opened too late for our Romac Reporters to write us about it, but this is what we know: The menu is World Fusion, served tapas style (small dishes, good for sharing among members of a group). The room is a mix of modern and deco elements: there's a glass block front wall, a large banquette across from the long bar, and exposed brick walls/hardwood floors. Jazz most nights.

Deux Cheminees

$60

1221 Locust St., Philadelphia (215) 790-0200
bet. 12th & 13th Sts. in Center City

This award-winning Classic French restaurant is "Paris on Locust Street." Chef/owner Fritz Blank is renowned for his "personable" approach, so you should expect a charming chat along with your "superb" meal, then perhaps a "fun" tour of his library of cookbooks. "Way to go, Fritz!"

Dickens Inn

$27

421 S. 2nd St., Philadelphia (215) 928-9307
bet. Pine & Lombard in the Historic Area

The "extraordinary atmosphere" that can only result from a British pub (with many authentic bric-a-brac) in a three story Federal Townhouse in Head House Square. While the food may only be rated "good," remember that it's British food. "Good" British food can mean "Beef Wellington that is out of this world" and very good shepherd's pie. Go for the bar, with its "excellent beers" and cozy fireplace. "One of my father's favorites," says one voter, but we don't know if that's a compliment or not.

Di Giovanni

$26

2500 S. Broad St., Philadelphia (215) 389-3121
at Porter St. in So. Phila.

The Roman and Regional Italian food is actually above average in most voters' opinion, at this South Broad establishment, in the heart of the Avenue of the Arts. A few grumblers bring the averages down, but that's to be expected for a place that gets busy before and after game time.

D'Ignazio's Towne House

$25

117 Veteran's Sq., Media (610) 566-6141
at Baltimore Pk. in Delaware County

The food may only be "fair," but it's always "very consistent" at this hulking behemoth in Media. Serving Italian and American food with seafood specialties, it has many amenities available to its 1,200 seats, from a fireplace to Jefferson Dining With Heart menu items, early bird specials and pipe and cigar smoking in the "Stag Bar." "A good place to take seniors."

= Superior = Excellent = Very Good

DiLullo Centro

$42

1407 Locust St., Philadelphia (215) 546-2000
bet. Broad & 15th in Center City

In the site of the old Locust Street Theater, hand-painted murals set the scene, and live music from the piano lounge adds an elegant touch. And while the ratings average "very good," the vote was split: what is "always a treat" to some is "highly overrated" to others. Preview it with the pre-orchestra bar food specials. If you like it, you can come back for the feature presentation.

Dilworthtown Inn

$41

1390 Old Wilmington Pk., West Chester (610) 399-1390
in Chester County

"Excellent, excellent, excellent" read the ratings of this "elegant," "lovely country inn." The "rustic" atmosphere, a bit more dressy since the fire renovation three years ago, has diners from all over donning their ties and evening dresses (separately, of course) and making the "way off" trek to West Chester. Clearly at the top of many voter's lists, they say it's "expensive, but worth it." P.S. Try the outdoor dining in the ruins of the c. 1700's stables.

DiMarco's

$27

16th & Ritner Sts., Philadelphia (215) 271-5117
in So. Phila.

Ten years of service to the South Philly Italian and Continental scene have not helped this mid-sized restaurant distinguish itself, at least in our ratings. Trying to appeal to everyone, the food may be a bit "bland" according to voters, though they like the Victorian motif, with handcrafted stained glass windows made by the DiMarcos themselves. Prices are on the high side for a family restaurant.

DiNardo's

$24

312 Race St., Philadelphia (215) 925-5115
bet. 3rd & 4th Sts. in the Historic Area

The Old City Seafood spot, No. 1 in the city for hard-shell crabs, is "always busy," so expect to wait for a table to taste "spicy and hot" crabs, "superb steamed mussels" and "great spicy French fries." Voters warn that "the rest of the fare is less alluring" and most think the room is dingy.

Dining Car & Market

$16

8826 Frankford Ave., Philadelphia (215) 338-5113
Frankford Ave. & Academy Rd. in Northeast Phila.

What? We've got a diner here! You'll get everything you'd expect from a diner at this 35-year-old Northeast Philly fixture: low prices, charmingly corny music, healthy menu options, a bottomless cup of Joe and a door that never closes. If this is everything you're looking for, this is a "great place," provided you're after food that's "not bad," and service that's often "rude."

FOOD ROOM STAFF COST

Dining Room at the Ritz-Carlton

$46

17th & Chestnut Sts., Liberty Place, Philadelphia (215) 563-1600 in Center City

The Ritz-Carlton has reserved the Dining Room's dinner hour for private functions only, but it's still open for breakfast and lunch, and is a contender for "the best brunch in the city." "Just phenomenal—service and food—the best" sums up the comments about this formal American/Continental. Put on your blue suit and take your best client to lunch.

Dinon's

$28

133 E. Gay St., West Chester (610) 430-3600
bet. Walnut & Matlack Sts. in Chester County

This "small and intimate BYOB" in West Chester might be only a year old, but it has already acquired a core group of devoted fans. Originally the old Clemente's, one of the partners moved that establishment across the street while the other reopened this space as Dinon's. The result—a "reasonable" price and a menu that "can be excellent."

Dmitri's

$22

795 S. 3rd St., Philadelphia (215) 625-0556
at Catherine St. in So. Phila.

Romac Reporters swoon over the Mediterranean seafood at this tiny Queen Village BYO, which earned a top 20 food rating, and placed 5th for Philadelphia's Favorites. But getting a taste of "the best seafood in town" isn't for the fainthearted—the no-reservation policy makes a two-hour wait common. Regulars either arrive before opening time or while away the wait in the bar across the street, thinking about the "delicious" grilled octopus and "wonderful *Cioppino.*" Some say the room's cramped bustle "gives it a New York feel," but the consensus is clear: "Expand already and take reservations!"

Dock Street Brewery

$21

2 Logan Sq., Phila. (215) 496-0413 (18th & Cherry in Center City)

One of the most frequented spots in our polling area, Dock Street is also one of our voters' favorites, most notably for bar food and the all-important, after-work drink. With "one of the longest bars in Philly," the house brewed beer "is great, but reserve a yard glass a year in advance." The music blares, the game room bustles, but the food is "like in England—blah!" If you are just after the food, however, they let you bring your own wine. That's weird, isn't it?

Donecker's

$29

333 N. State St., Ephrata (717) 738-9501
at Walnut St. in Lancaster County

This is one of the more sophisticated dining and bed & breakfast options when you're far afield in Dutch Country. Owner William Donecker has organized an "excellent" staff and "very good" kitchen under one elegant, "romantic" roof, that includes lovely hotel rooms. The Classic French cuisine is complemented by a large wine selection, many available by the glass, and special attention to lighter, healthier options, with an emphasis on fresh, local ingredients.

 = Superior = Excellent = Very Good

Dori Italian

$26

900 N. Bethlehem Pk., Spring House (215) 646-6116
Norristown & Tennis in Montgomery County

Start with a slightly-above average, "very traditional Italian" menu, then start adding features and you've got this well frequented spot in Springhouse. The "old classics are done well," with "giant" portions to boot, especially during the "great early bird special." Add to that an elegant setting, with a dance floor and a piano bar with a sing-a-long, and you have a "solid performer."

Downey's

$27

Front & South Sts., Phila. (215) 625-9500 (in the South St. Area)

Plenty of people like to visit this "classic neighborhood Irish pub," with its "friendly crowd of all ages," but typically, it's not for the food, which only earns "fair" to "good" marks. It's the "great bar," and group-oriented activities like singalongs, that attract the after-work crowd, who watch South Street go by from the veranda.

Down Home Diner

$12

12th & Filbert Sts., Reading Terminal Market, Philadelphia
(215) 627-1955 (in Center City)

"Carolina cookin' in Philly! Mmmmmmm!" articulates one reviewer, though owner Jack McDavid, of Jack's Firehouse, would have you believe that the '50s diner food has been updated with "fresh, '90s ingredients." This is a diner, remember, so the "breakfasts are to die for," or, in one voter's opinion, are "the best hangover food."

Down Home Grill

$12

1800 Spring Garden St., Philadelphia (215) 557-7510
at 18th St. in the Art Museum Area

Two things distinguish this Jack McDavid offering from his other two restaurants: a "non-descript," "banal environment," and low food scores. Stick with the Down Home Diner.

Drafting Room

$21

635 N. Pottstown Pk., Exton (610) 363-0521
Ship Rd. & Rt. 100 on the Main Line

While this Exton Multiethnic Contemporary is named for the room, the food and the staff ratings beat it by a good margin. And that speaks well of the food, as do our voters: the "innovative menu," created by chefs recently acquired from other restaurants, has "great food at a great price." Here's a yearling that is "up and coming."

Drexel Ale House

$17

State Rd. and Lansdowne Ave., Bond Shopping Ctr., Upper Darby
(610) 789-9833 (in Delaware County)

We hear there's a big staff turnover at this Upper Darby American, and that the owner spends much of his time trying to whip things into shape. But what aspires to an eclectic menu, with fish and other grill choices, still remains a destination for simpler fare for our voters. "A nice place for a drink and conversation."

FOOD ROOM STAFF COST

Duling-Kurtz

$40

146 S. Whitford Rd., Exton (610) 524-1830 at Rt. 30 on the Main Line

Our voters rave more about the "enchanting," "romantic fireplace rooms" and the "beautiful gardens" than about the "good" and "unusual food" at this Exton American. A "special occasion place," with a large selection of wines by the glass, remember to call ahead if you want a seat. And no, two guys named Kurt don't come out and face off during dinner.

Eagle Tavern

$25

Rt. 100, Eagle (610) 458-5331 (in Chester County)

There's nothing pretentious about this cozy, casual spot in Chester County, where Romac Reporters find "a very relaxed atmosphere" and "good bar food." Older voters say it's "the best food for the money," while younger ones appreciate the "very nice people" at this "historic working man's tavern where you will feel at home."

East Side Mario's

$17

180 Old Lincoln Hwy., Exton (610) 363-0444
at Rt. 100 on the Main Line

This Exton chain Italian takes atmosphere to movie set extremes—the place is done up like a Depression-era Little Italy streetside cafe, complete with storefronts. Voters like the "boisterous, friendly" staff and "fun atmosphere," and say the food is "tasty and inexpensive." You can take kids, but the restaurant won't take reservations.

Elephant & Castle at the Holiday Inn Center City

$18

18th & Market Sts., Philadelphia (215) 751-9977 (in Center City)

The British-style pub grub doesn't get passing marks from Romac Reporters, who say the "menu is limited and food wasn't as good as I expected." They like the room, which features darts and pubby decor, but the service grades are only fair.

Ellen Rose Restaurant

$25

5920 Greene St., Phila. (215) 843-1525 (Haines St. in Germantown)

What started as a Georgian-style home in 1892 has become a local favorite in Germantown. Chef/owner Ellen Appelbaum prepares an eclectic International menu that earns above average marks from the under 30 crowd (who might not be used to good home cooking), and good marks from everyone else. A cozy setting, "nice owners," a lovely garden for dining outside in nice weather and reasonable prices make diners feel like welcome guests in a gracious home.

Engine 46

VOTE

Reed & Water Sts., Philadelphia (215) 462-4646 (in So. Phila.)

A late night menu (served until 2 a.m.), kid-friendliness (kids' menu, free fire hats), and other firehouse-related items are what you'd expect from a mid-priced family-oriented steakhouse, located in an old fire station. What you might not expect are tablecloths patterned after dalmation spots: check it out, and let us know on your questionnaire if this new local is destined for chaindom.

 = Superior = Excellent = Very Good

Epicurean $24

902 Village at Eland, Rt. 113, Phoenixville (610) 933-1336
at Dawson Dr. in Chester County

Our reviewers recommend chef/owner Lee Krasley's mid-sized, mid-priced, and average-looking bar/restaurant for one reason—or should we say 200 reasons. That's the size of his "vast beer collection," including some international rarities and seasonal brews. These are complemented by "creative appetizers and bar foods," but voters say you should keep it simple and stay away from the "heavy entrees."

Erin Pub $18

36 W. Winons Ave., Norwood (610) 461-0991
at Chester Pk. in Delaware County

What sounds like an Irish Pub is really a "very good" American, with so many fans that, although it accomodates 200, "there isn't enough seating." It's a "great place for lobster and prime rib... the best and inexpensive!" You will find the Irish flavor in the live music Friday and Saturday nights, (Irish dance lessons between sets), and in the variety of "good imported beers."

Essene Cafe $18

719 S. 4th St., Philadelphia (215) 928-3722
at Monroe St. in So. Phila.

"Delicious" food that's also "good for you?" Must be the high-quality, fresh organic ingredients that go into the menu at this charming little Vegetarian and fish restaurant in South Philly. Of course there's no smoking, but you can get a little unhealthy by bringing your own wine or beer, if you wish. Oh, and they also serve espresso, though health-conscious diners usually opt for the fresh organic juice bar.

Evermay-on-the-Delaware $53

River Rd., Erwinna (610) 294-9100
at Headquarters Rd. in Bucks County

If you're planning on antiquing through Bucks County, are looking for a "great weekend getaway" (the hotel is nestled in 25 acres of gardens and woodland paths), or you just want an "excellent" prix fixe meal (the menu is "limited, but an exceptional value"), call well in advance to this Contemporary American, and reserve a table in the historic dining room. Here is a place where fresh ingredients are paramount, complemented by a very good wine list. Dress up, but wear comfortable shoes to stroll around the lovely grounds.

Fairmount Bagel Institute $7

267 S. 19th St., Phila. (215) 735-2222 at Rittenhouse Sq. in Ctr. City
2501 Olive St., Philadelphia (215) 235-2245 in the Art Museum Area

What have our voters learned at this Institute of Low Price? For starters, go there for the "best bagels in the city— chewy and cheap!" With "jillions" (technical term) of different kinds of flavored cream cheese, FBI is even doing its part to rejuvenate the city: "We may never leave Philly because of the salmon spread."

FOOD ROOM STAFF COST

Family Chen

$17

4341 Main St., Philadelphia (215) 483-2050 in Manayunk/Roxborough

Some reviewers say "Manayunk still needs a decent Chinese restaurant," while others argue that this fits the requirements—"very nice people" and "some good choices," especially dishes like salmon in black bean sauce and Grandpa's bean curd. The best advice: "Stick with the basics."

Famous 4th St. Deli

$11

700 S. 4th St., Philadelphia (215) 922-3274 at Bainbridge St. in the South St. Area

Comments and votes are all over the map for this Queen Village Traditional Jewish Deli, from a large group of voters. Open seven days a week for breakfast and brunch, its fans appreciate the good smoked fish and corned beef, but detractors say it's a little "cramped," so you should only "go for the history." All disagreements aside, sharpen your sweet tooth and save room, the chocolate chip cookies are "to DIE for," and may well be the "best in Philly."

Felicia's

$30

1148 S. 11th St., Philadelphia (215) 755-9656 at Ellsworth St. in So. Phila.

Fans, and there are plenty, of this small South Philly Northern Italian rave about the "best restaurant in South Philly," with "the best gnocci... ever," and "no better stuffed pork chops anywhere else." Such popularity in a small restaurant leads some to complain it can be "crowded" and "smoky and noisy."

Felicia's Pizza Kitchen

$12

18 W. Lancaster Ave., Ardmore (610) 649-6900 on the Main Line

You'll notice it's not called "Felicia's Pizza Kitchen and dining room." That's because this traditional brick-oven pizzeria in Ardmore is takeout only, though next spring promises a new deck and tables. It's "upscale pizza, for sure," says one voter, and other comments range from "consistently good takeout" to "the best pizza around!"

Fez Moroccan

$26

620 S. 2nd St., Philadelphia (215) 925-5367 bet. South & Bainbridge in the South St. Area

Like most Moroccan restaurants, this Queen Village storefront offers a complete feast for the price of an entree at many restaurants—eight courses for $20. Diners recline on sofas around a brass table, while belly dancers entertain between courses. Reviewers call it "a fun group dining experience." Reservations are essential.

 = Superior = Excellent = Very Good

Fiddler's Green

$22

208 W. Beidler Rd., Sweetbriar Square Shopping Ctr, King of Prussia (610) 337-3888
at N. Henderson Rd. in Montgomery County

Owner Joe Hindlsey makes this friendly Irish pub with American food a "fun place for a group," especially when he belts out show tunes and traditional Irish songs on weekend nights. With "good food, at a good value," order a drink and some corned beef and cabbage, and get in the mood. One crabby customer thinks "you have to be Irish."

1521 Cafe Gallery

VOTE

1521 Spruce St., Philadelphia (215) 546-1521
bet. 15th & 16th in Center City

This light fare restaurant in Center City has found a way to start small, and never disappoint its customers in the process. It began as an art gallery, and remains one, providing a unique and "great" environment to meet and chat. Then they added coffee and dessert, which they do very well, right down to the little chocolates. Finally, they added "very good" though "limited" light fare, creating a place that "could be pretentiously hip," but has "too much of a mom-and-pop feel" to ever get that way.

Fingers

$26

700 Bethlehem Pk., Erdenheim (215) 233-9955
in Montgomery County

Although the chef was trained at London's Dorcester Hotel, the food earns only so-so marks at this Erdenheim Continental. Still, many regulars frequent this place, for the friendly atmosphere that includes a singalong at the piano bar, and for the many specials. Wednesdays, all lunch entrees are $5, and on any Sunday when the Eagles win, dinner entrees are reduced to $10 each.

Flanigan's Boat House

$16

113 Fayette St., Conshohocken (610) 828-2628 (828-BOAT)
bet. 1st & 2nd in Montgomery County

The food is "good," if unspectacular at this Conshohocken American. But the atmosphere, with plenty of singles, families, and other locals, who stop by for "great wings," or "a drink after softball," is what hauls them into the Boat House. It's a little too "noisy and smoky" for some, but if you like a wide selection of beers, row on over.

Flowing Springs Inn

$31

Rt. 100, Spring City (610) 469-0899
bet. Rts. 23 & 401 in Chester County

If it weren't for the very good room and ambiance rating, we would think twice about including this so-so Continental in our book. The food is called everything from "boring" to "fair," with unspectacular service to match. If you want "elegant atmosphere," or a stay at the bed and breakfast, this is your place.

FOOD ROOM STAFF COST

Flying Fish

$31

8142 Germantown Ave., Philadelphia (215) 247-0707
at Hartwell Ln. in Chestnut Hill/Mt. Airy

With "fantastic fish and atmosphere" Paul Roller's seafood restaurant in Chestnut Hill, though sometimes "noisy," is a "good date restaurant," has a kids' menu, and welcomes parents with infants. The interior has a very clean look, with linen on the tables and local artists on the walls, but some ask "could they get the tables any closer?"

Foggia

$21

24th & Lombard Sts., Philadelphia (215) 731-9424 in Center City

A few voters are happy to report that this year-old, Center City Northern Italian is an "excellent new restaurant in a location that has been the kiss of death for many predecessors." Others are not so impressed. The staff, especially for a relatively new place, is great, called "friendly" and professional. Reviewers also advise you "ask for a table on the top floor."

Forager

VOTE

1600 River Rd., New Hope (215) 862-9477 in Bucks County

The huge oil painting, depicting the view from the tower in New Hope, is what you see when you enter. The very good American/International cuisine is what you remember after you leave. Brick oven pizza, grilled specialities and special prix fixes on Mondays and Thursdays are of "consistently high quality"—and the "nice people" who work there help to make it one of our voters' "all-time favorites."

Founders at the Bellevue Hotel

$48

1415 Chancellor Ct., Philadelphia (215) 790-2814
Broad & Walnut in Center City

Our voters give top marks to the room and the staff of this "elegant," usually "excellent" American/Continental restaurant, with lovely 19th floor views from atop the Bellevue in Center City. While one diner recommends it as "an elegant place for an out-of-town guest," Philadelphians also treasure it as one of the "only romantic spots for dining and dancing." Call ahead to reserve, and keep it in mind for a private party off "one of the most beautiful dining rooms anywhere."

Fountain at the Four Seasons

$56

One Logan Sq., Philadelphia (215) 963-1500
18th & Ben Franklin Pkwy. in Center City

The top overall restaurant on our poll, the Fountain is also in many of our Top 10 lists: You'll find it all over the front of the book. Page after page of voters' comments simply glow about this fabulous French/Continental: "Spectacular in every way," "consistently the best in the city," "the best anywhere," "never a mistake, always perfect"—you get the picture. Sunday brunch is a standout, called "an epicurean feast," and we suggest you reserve for Mother's Day a year in advance.

 = Superior = Excellent = Very Good

Fragrant Chives

$30

1623 Walnut St., Phila. (215) 563-7776 bet. 16th & 17th in Ctr. City

This elegant new entry to the Walnut Street dining scene has not yet caught on with many Romac Reporters. The few who have visited give Fragrant Chives their highest ratings. Can Walnut Street support another upscale Chinese? Tell us on your questionnaire.

Frankie's Seafood Italiano

$28

1100 Tasker St., Phila. (215) 468-9989 (at 11th St. in So. Phila.)

There are arguments over whether the Italian seafood at this South Philly neighborhood spot is "great" or not, but everyone agrees there's "plenty of it." They always cook to order, except at the oyster bar. Check it out before a game, or give them a call—this place is "packed on weekends."

Frederick's

VOTE

757 S. Front St., Philadelphia (215) 271-3733 (in So. Phila.)

Nearly brand-new on Front Street, this little Regional Italian is rapidly becoming a popular pick, particularly for the appetizer, salad and antipasto push cart they wheel from table to table during late night. The "very good," charming and nostalgic atmosphere includes a 100-year-old bar and a view of the park. If you have a wait, relax—"Dave the bartender is the best."

Fresh Fields Cafe

$10

821 Lancaster Ave., Devon (610) 688-9400 (on the Main Line)

"Thank heaven for Fresh Fields," writes one health nut, it's "healthy and good!" While they supply fresh produce, juices and the like, their sandwiches, "great wheatless cakes" and other "yuppified deli and cafe" items are great for takeout, or for the little tables outside when the weather's nice. One pre-food pyramid holdout groans "too healthy—tastes too much like grains."

Friday's

$18

4000 City Line Ave., Phila. (215) 878-7070 in the City Line Area
Oxford Valley Mall, Langhorne (215) 750-8002 (in Bucks County)
King of Prussia Plaza, King of Prussia (610) 768-9340 in Montgomery County
17th & J.F.K. Pkwy., Phila. (215) 665-8443 (in Center City)
2nd & Lombard Sts., Phila. (215) 625-8389 (in South St. Area)
Willow Grove Mall, Willow Grove (215) 657-1597 in Montgomery County

Ignore the food rating and focus on the many honor spots this chain occupies in the front of our book. It is number 1 for bar food, number 3 for after-work drinks and children (does one lead to the other?) and is in the top 10 for eavesdropping and even vegetarian menus. So what's the attraction? Most see it as a "run-of-the-mill singles restaurant," though admit the burgers and sandwiches are pretty good. Who knows? Someday this may be the only place to go for fried cheese.

FOOD ROOM STAFF COST

Friday, Saturday, Sunday $27

261 S. 21st St., Phila. (215) 546-4232
bet. Locust & Spruce in Center City
Despite a fraction of Monday Morning naysayers, this "romantic," cozy little Continental and American in Center City has nothing but fans. "The fish tank is awesome," and is a highlight to an otherwise "great room," that is usually "very crowded and NOISY!" "A great date place," and "reasonable," "there's a good chance of running into someone famous." Like who, Tuesday Weld?

Fuji Mountain $29

2030 Chestnut St., Phila. (215) 751-0939 (at 21st St. in Center City)
A newcomer to Center City, many overlook this Japanese simply because it is on the second floor. It is bigger than most Japanese restaurants in the area, literally—they don't cram the tables in, so it has a more open, if somewhat more impersonal feel. The tatami rooms have paper walls, so they don't drown out the Karaoke coming from the third floor.

Fuji Mountain $28

801 Montgomery Ave., Narberth (610) 668-9959 (on the Main Line)
The locals call this Narberth Japanese "a nice addition to the area," even if it is "a little cramped and noisy." Other voters aren't so nice. One rake asserts this joint "should have stayed a gas station," while another simply calls the staff "rude." On the constructive side, one voter offers that it "would be better if the staff could understand you."

Gallo Nero

VOTE

504 E. Bethlehem Pk., Ambler (215) 654-5000 (Montgomery Cty.)
Il Gallo Nero has changed its name to Ristorante Gallo Nero, and moved to an old schoolhouse at the side of the road in Springhouse. Owners Enzo and Carla Fusaro are just completing renovations at the time this book goes to print— let us know what you think on your questionnaire next year.

Garden $40

1617 Spruce St., Phila. (215) 546-4455 (bet. 15th & 16th in Ctr. City)
Not your garden-variety American and Continental restaurant, this superb Center City spot, in an historic building (1870), has more seating outside than in: both settings are called "beautiful," and it wins our Top 10 for outdoor dining. Pick a night when the weather isn't too forbidding, and you're in store for a very pleasant, "romantic" evening. The Garden also places high in our business dinner category. One of Philly's favorites, reserve well in advance.

Garnian Wa $14

1776 E. Rt. 30, Paoli Plaza, Paoli (610) 889-1761 on the Main Line
With a chef/owner named Hung Chow Chau, it has to be good Chinese, brought to you by the same management as the Sampan Inn in Havertown. It's a good suburban Chinese, with few standouts besides "fast service," in a Westernized decor.

Gas Light

$18

100 E. Hinckley Ave., across from Ridley Park Train Sta., Ridley Park (610) 521-9060 (at Sellers Ave. in Delaware County)

This little Continental in Ridley Park harkens back to Victorian England, when the rooms were small, and, unfortunately, the food wasn't all that spectacular. However, with limited seating, and a good staff, there are always lines at this "cozy and friendly spot." Call ahead and see if you can get a seat on the porch in nice weather.

General Warren Inne

$35

W. Old Lancaster Hwy., Malvern (610) 296-3637
at Rt. 29 on the Main Line

This recently restored historic Malvern Continental gets very good marks for its traditional menu with contemporary specials and "charming" dining room with three working fireplaces. The service also gets very good grades—tableside dishes are a specialty. Add an extensive wine list and "delicious desserts" and it's clear why some call it "the best restaurant in the Main Line area."

Genji I & II

$25

4002 Spruce St., Philadelphia (215) 387-1583
at 40th St. in University City/W. Phila.
1720 Sansom St., Philadelphia (215) 564-1720
bet. 17th & 18th Sts. in Center City

"I'd spend my trust fund on sushi at this place," writes one reviewer, and many others are happy enough just to eat "the best sushi in the city." With a food rating in the Top 100, while it is "unusually good," it is also "quick." It may well be the "best you've ever had," in Philadelphia or anywhere else. For you folks who like your food cooked, Genji has many other very good Japanese options on the menu.

Geno's Steaks

$8

9th St. & Passyunk Ave., Philadelphia (no phone)(in So. Phila.)

Holding the line against Pat's (right across the street) in the endless and sometimes bloody (but certainly, always greasy) Philly cheesesteak war, Geno's places a close third in our book for best cheesesteak in town. And we all know what that means. At 2:00am, you'll find an assortment of cholesterol junkies, in various states of consciousness, standing in line under the flourescent lights or huddled over their steaks at the outdoor picnic tables (the only seating) for warmth. "With Pat's across the street, why bother?" asks one voter. Some people just go for the glamor, we guess.

Genuardi Food Court

$10

550 E. Lancaster Ave., St. David's Sq., St. Davids (610) 989-0759
on the Main Line

"How could you include this place in a serious survey" asks one reviewer of these prepared food and salad bar takeout spots, located in Genuardi's supermarket. Well, throngs of voters wouldn't miss it, for while "it's hard to rave, it's fun for a quick meal." An easy "lunch spot," this "good fast food" also fits the bill for work-weary parents: "It's our kids' favorite place to eat."

FOOD ROOM STAFF COST

Georgine's

$27

1320 Newport Rd., West Bristol (215) 785-0564
Rts. 413 & 13 in Bucks County

You get Texas-size seafood and steaks at this Bucks County American, and our voters agree that "you'll never leave hungry." Unfortunately, "Georgine's practice of not taking reservations can mean up to a three-hour wait on weekends. That's a long time at the bar!" Oh, and here's something you don't often hear in Bucks County: "too glitzy."

Gillane's Tavern

$18

43 Cricket Ave., Ardmore (610) 896-1622
at Lancaster Ave. on the Main Line

This Ardmore American serves everything from "Philly's best turkey sandwich" and cheesesteaks at the bar to surf and turf in the dining room, where green leather booths hark back to Prohibition-era roots.

Girasole

$29

1305 Locust St., Philadelphia (215) 985-4659
bet. 13th & Broad in Center City

It is an attractive place, with terracotta floors, fresh flowers, and a simple, country Italian design, but that doesn't keep our voters from disagreeing about the regional Italian menu. Some call it "good food," citing the "excellent pizza" made from "simple, fresh ingredients." Others find the portions small, calling Girasole "overpriced," and not without its staffing problems.

Giuseppe's Pizza

$11

46 S. Bethlehem Pk., Ambler (215) 628-4616 (Montgomery Cty.)

Where else but a pizza joint do you find a good food rating with such lousy room and staff ratings? Close your eyes, and order one of their "excellent pizzas," in what our kinder voters call "a no-frills establishment." "Garlic pizza reigns!"

Goat Hollow

$22

300 W. Mt. Pleasant Ave., Philadelphia (215) 242-4710
at Lincoln Dr. in Chestnut Hill/Mt. Airy

"The parking is sometimes a challenge" at this dark, brass-and-candle American in Mt. Airy, "but the food is well worth it!" The "great bar" and dining room is populated by a "friendly crowd" of regulars, who come for the food and linger for the live country, rock or blues. Don't worry, the restaurant's namesake isn't on the menu.

Golden Pheasant Inn

$45

763 River Rd., Erwinna (610) 294-9595
in Bucks County

Between the Delaware River and the Pennsylvania Canal, you'll find this 1857 fieldstone inn, serving very good Classic French food in three cozy dining rooms. Chef/owner Michel Faure and wife Barbara have created one of the top "Sleepers" in our book. If you've got that "big date," go here, and bear in mind that the inn also has elegant rooms with four-poster canopy beds and lovely views.

Golden Pond Chinese

$20

1006 Race St., Phila. (215) 923-0303 (bet. 10th & 11th in Chinatown)
The ingredients are fresh, the menu options healthy, even the water is filtered at this "excellent" Chinese restaurant in Chinatown. Run by a "lovely family," the service is among the highest rated in the book. But they really distinguish themselves with their food, voted one of the top vegetarians in the city.

Golden Sea

VOTE

Rts. 202 & 73, Clover Mall, Centre Square (610) 292-8881 in Montgomery Co.
Folks think highly of this Centre Square Chinese, which serves Cantonese, Hunan and Szechuan specialties. The decor is above average, and way above average for Chinese, even if it's not to everyone's taste. You can always take out, but we hear the "ginger salmon is the best," so you might want to eat in and order seconds.

Goodnoe Farm Dairy Bar

$12

Rt. 532, Newtown (215) 968-3875 in Bucks County
"Limit your visits to ice cream, and you'll be very pleased," say our voters of this Newtown ice-cream-parlor-cum-restaurant. The "great ice cream" is made fresh, though there may be "too many high school kids there on Saturday night." As for the food—fair, yes. Good? No.

Gourmet Restaurant

$33

3520 Cottman Ave., Phila. (215) 331-7174 (Frankford Ave. in NE Phila.)
A few of our voters came through, and gave us the skinny on this "very good" French restaurant in the Northeast. The Thai heritage of the owners is reflected in some unusual preparations of familiar French dishes, and always with great results. Start with the "best cucumber soup" and go on to the "best lamb chops," and don't worry, it isn't as pricey as comparable French restaurants in Center City.

Gracie's 21st C. Cafe

$40

Manatawny Rd., Pine Forge (610) 323-4004 in Berks County
One of the top Sleepers on our poll, this Eclectic little spot really pulled down the big numbers, especially for Pine Forge, prompting one voter to call it "a delightful jewel in a dining wilderness." In case they're putting together a brochure, another reviewer offers that it's "a mini-vacation to the Mediterranean—mind, body and spirit are refreshed." Well, you might need that kind of rejuvenation after the "long drive," but the "excellent" fare is well worth it. This is a real find.

Grasshopper

$28

4427 Main St., Phila. (215) 483-1888 at Carson St. in Manayunk/Roxborough
French and Chinese cuisines prove a winning combination at this smallish Manayunk spot. Most voters, conservative with their numerical ratings, state that "the food is excellent and the owner is very pleasant." While a few grumblers hate to face the fact that "the prices keep rising," the BYO policy keeps it a good value.

= Good **= Fair** **[no rating] = Poor**

FOOD ROOM STAFF COST

Gravina

$25

1710-12 Grant Ave., Philadelphia (215) 969-6275
at Bustleton Ave. in Northeast Phila.

Voters say this Northeast Philadelphia Italian serves "consistently good pizzas and entrees from the wood-fired oven" in an atmosphere that owes less to the decor than to the background music: all the great Italian singers from—you guessed it—Pavarotti to Sinatra.

Great American Grill

$18

Rt. 611 & Rt. 32, Kintnersville (610) 847-2023 (in Bucks County)

This Montgomery County Regional American has a lot of country charm, from its setting on 22 acres of woods and fields to the home-smoke foods (try the all-you-can-eat rib special on weeknights). The restaurant caters to kids by covering all the tables with white paper and supplying crayons; the best results decorate the walls. It has an extensive beer list that changes seasonally.

Greeks

$16

239 Haverford Ave., Narberth (610) 664-8655
at Narberth Ave. on the Main Line

The Greeks at this Narberth Tavern are more of the fraternity kind, who would rather chase you a beer than a salad with olives and feta. "What a surprise to find such great food in a bar," says one of the American food, owing to a recent change of ownership and a change in the kitchen.

Green Hills Inn

$40

2444 Morgantown Rd., Reading (610) 777-9611 (in Berks County)

"Do yourself a favor—take the drive and go" to Reading, for simply "excellent" French/American fare. Chef/owner Jay Schaeffer attends to all the details: The cordial, professional staff, the wine list with an emphasis on good values, and the fresh country ingredients in the somewhat Provençal menu have propelled this out-of-the -way place to near the top of our Sleepers list.

Grill & Bar at the Ritz-Carlton

$43

17th & Chestnut Sts., Liberty Pl., Phila. (215) 563-1600 (Ctr. City)

One of the survey's top spots for food—some say "the second-best in the city"—and a "great hangout bar" make the Grill & Bar the choice when you're in the mood for "the best of everything" and don't mind paying for it. The room is formal—both jackets and reservations are required—but the "personable staff" and "excellent food" make it a place Romac Reporters "highly recommend."

Gullifty's

$18

1149 Lancaster Ave., Rosemont (610) 525-1851 (on the Main Line)

The ratings may only be fair-to-middling, but the portions are big and the prices low at this Rosemont Eclectic. Even the rooms are eclectic, with a Pub, a clubby room downstairs, and an airy, outdoorsy room upstairs. Romac Reporters love the staff, but some warn that the clientele sometimes parties too much.

= Superior = Excellent = Very Good

Gypsie Rose $29

505 Bridge Rd., Collegeville (610) 489-1600
Rt. 113, just N. of Rt. 29 in Montgomery County

Stripped to its essentials, the 18th-century building and its creekside setting are the come-ons at this Collegeville American Regional. "Watching the stream roll by" creates a romantic atmosphere for such dishes as Maryland crab cakes and Chicken Philadelphia. Despite "friendly owners," though, some voters wonder, "what service?"

Hacienda $30

36 W. Mechanic St., New Hope (215) 862-2078
at New St. in Bucks County

This Continental has been pampering New Hope's theater audiences since the '60s with traditional seafood and beef dishes. Voters say the art deco decor "seems a little outdated," but find the prices "reasonable for New Hope." Among its other selling points: prix fixe dinners, a pianist on weekends, a nice view of the village and proximity to the playhouse.

Hadley's at the Sheraton Society Hill $32

1 Dock St., Philadelphia (215) 238-6656
near 2nd & Walnut in the Historic Area

This Historic Area Hotel American (with European influences) isn't exactly up to what you might expect from hotel dining. The food, while sometimes "innovative," earns only average marks, with portions shrinking lately according to some. But the place has a solid, comfortable feel, and Hadley's is not up to the usual pretension and price of most other hotel restaurants.

Hana Japanese $23

387 Lancaster Ave., Strafford Shopping Ctr., Wayne
(610) 687-3320 at Conestoga Rd. on the Main Line

Just when our voters thought this Japanese in Wayne had "slipped over the years," Chef Yori Shima returned from his sushi restaurant in Japan to reclaim the title of "best sushi chef in the area." Still, "non-descript" decor and the "little variety" on the menu make some diners think twice about eating in, and an above-average price tag, especially for a suburban ethnic BYO, makes others think twice about taking out.

H & J McNally's Tavern $16

8634 Germantown Ave., Philadelphia (215) 247-9736
Bethlehem Pk. in Chestnut Hill/Mt. Airy

Lots of places serve good sandwiches and beer on tap, but only this Chestnut Hill pub rests its reputation on the Schmitter, a cheesesteak with fried onions, salami and a secret sauce. Locals like the Harp on tap, served in 20 oz. glasses, "great soup and sammies," and the "nice" neighborhood tavern ambiance.

FOOD ROOM STAFF COST

Hank's Place

$11

Rts. 1 & 100, Chadds Ford (610) 388-7061 (in Delaware Cty.)
Scores for this American Diner in Chadds Ford are uncommonly extreme—voters are just as likely to say excellent or poor as good or very good. Its fans agree that breakfast and lunch are its best meals and praise the blueberry pancakes and fancy egg dishes. Dinner features "very traditional home cooking, like grandma used to make." It's a popular local hangout which, in these parts, means you might be seated next to one of the members of the local art community whose works hang on the walls—maybe even a Wyeth!

Happy Rooster

$37

118 S. 16th St., Philadelphia (215) 563-1481
at Sansom St. in Center City
All crowing cock jokes aside, our voters advise that this little Continental/American in Center City, with its "well-stocked bar," is strictly "for the boys." "Don't bring a first date, if you want a second" advises one reviewer, and another warns "you won't be a happy rooster when you get the check."

Hardshell Cafe

$24

9th & Market Sts., Gallery at Market East, Philadelphia
(215) 592-9110 in Center City
355 York Rd., Warminster (215) 674-0600
bet. Street & County Line Rds. in Bucks County
You'll have to come out of your shell to get into this roll-up-your-sleeves, put-on-a-bib, and smash-it-with-a-mallet Seafood restaurant, specializing in, what else, crabs. But remember, this is Center City, not the shores of the Chesapeake, so be prepared for "pricey," if "awesome" food. "Their garlic style crabs are to die for!"

Harmony Vegetarian

$17

135 N. 9th St., Philadelphia (215) 627-4520
bet. Race & Cherry Sts. in Chinatown
One of the Top 10 Favorite Vegetarian restaurants in the city, they fool the eye, if not the palate, with faux-meat kosher Chinese dishes. What makes it the "best vegetarian" to some is the "largest selection," but others gripe that "gluten cannot taste like shrimp." Well, gluten can't clog up those arteries, either, and, despite a healthy reputation, Harmony is popular with kids.

Harry's Bar & Grill

$45

22 S. 18th St., Philadelphia (215) 561-5757
bet. Market & Chestnut in Center City
This "cozy little restaurant and bar" has become more casual since a renovation on the first floor, and the introduction of a new oyster bar. That doesn't stop it from being "the ultimate power lunch" in some voters' opinions, which translates into "good food, at high prices" to those who dine without the benefit of an expense account. The "old world ambiance" makes it "perfect for a quiet evening," dining on "the best petit filet in town."

 = Superior **= Excellent** **= Very Good**

Havana

$22

105 S. Main St., New Hope (215) 862-9897 in Bucks County
Not named for the food (Regional American), this place probably takes its name from the ambiance, called "very loud with too much smoking." "Fun and interesting," the food may only be average, but it's "inexpensive," and they have a "great deck on the street in the summer." The historic building belies a kid-friendly, family setting.

Herb Garden Cafe

$26

19 S. Whitehorse Rd., Phoenixville (610) 935-5988
at Rt. 23 in Chester County
This Eclectic Victorian in Phoenixville recently added a deck so patrons can enjoy a view of the herb gardens while they sip their own wine. The herbs end up in "tasty and inventive food" from a kitchen that "does a great job for a small, out of the way place." Voters love the prices, the specials and details like flavored coffees, but are less impressed with the service and decor. Live jazz occasionally.

Hikaru

$26

4348 Main St., Philadelphia (215) 487-3500
at Grape St. in Manayunk/Roxborough
607 S. 2nd St., Philadelphia (215) 627-7110 in the South St. Area
108 S. 18th St., Philadelphia (215) 496-9950 in Center City
Our voters are evenly mixed about the food at these traditional Japanese spots, probably since its most popular Manayunk location is little more than two years old. You can't argue with "very clean" and "good presentation" when it comes to sushi, or Teppan-Yaki, cooked right at your table. When asked about sushi, someone inevitably says it's "overpriced:" Most agree Hikaru has "good sushi" at "reasonable prices."

Hoa Viet

$13

1022 Race St., Philadelphia (215) 592-8540
bet. 10th & 11th in Chinatown
The "good menu, and reasonable prices" are reason enough to visit this Chinatown Chinese and Vietnamese, but the "spectacular number of choices" and the fact that they can accommodate groups of up to 10 give it something of an edge over neighboring spots. Even with a big group, you'll never be able to sample everything here.

Hog Island Foods

VOTE

11th & Walnut Sts., Philadelphia (215) 627-7511
in the Historic Area
This deli is too new to have caught on with many Romac Reporters. Those who have visited say the owner "cares about the food:" he recreates the hoagie's progenitor, the hogie, a filled loaf that is prepared by mixing (Caesar Salad-style) meats, lettuce, roasted peppers, and other goodies, and stuffing them into a hollowed-out roll. We hope next year's voters will tell us who deserves the "A"—the hogie or the hoagie.

FOOD ROOM STAFF COST

Ho Sai Gai

$17

10th & Race Sts., Philadelphia (215) 922-5883 in Chinatown

The room rating is the only one that held its ground over last year, and that's not saying much. The price has gone up, as our voters' opinions of the food has come down. Still, it has the location and the hours (open til 4-5 a.m. daily), though one diner advises "only if every other restaurant in Chinatown has a long wait."

Hotel Du Village

VOTE

N. River & Phillips Mill Rds., New Hope (215) 862-9911 in Bucks Co.

This Country French occupies a historic Tudor-style building on 10 landscaped acres in New Hope. Voters who have discovered its peaceful setting and "always gracious" chef/owners simply say "excellent."

Houlihan's

$18

817 Old York Rd., Jenkintown (215) 887-6522 (in Mont. Co.)
225 S. 18th St., Philadelphia (215) 546-5940 in (Center City)
2250 E. Lincoln Hwy., Langhorne (215) 752-0110 (in Bucks Co.)
555 City Ave., Bala Cynwyd (610) 667-9717 (in City Line Area)
910 E. Woodland Ave., Springfield (610) 544-0200 in (Del. Co.)
Court at K. of Prussia, K. of Prussia (610) 337-9522 (in Mont. Co.)
601 W. Germantown Pk., Plymouth Meeting (610) 825-2537 in Montgomery County

What to some is a great singles scene with great bar fare, is to others "chain food" in a "jazzed-up meat market." The concensus? "A good plastic place, slightly better than the competition."

House of Hunan

$15

188 W. De Kalb Pk., Valley Forge Shopping Ctr., King of Prussia (610) 337-3950 in Montgomery County

If you're out by the Mall of Shopping, and can't think of anything better, or if you just want that sweet and salty Hunan brown sauce fix, drop by this serviceable, if no better than average Chinese restaurant. Its best features are the lunch buffet, and a separate room for non-smokers.

Hu-nan

$18

47 E. Lancaster Ave., Ardmore (610) 642-3050 at Rittenhouse Pl. on the Main Line

A few reviewers say this 20-year-old Ardmore Chinese makes "the best vegetable moo shoo, even better than in Chinatown." Healthy Hunan dishes are among the specialties. Others call it "overpriced" and think "the food has gone downhill."

Hugo's Inn

$20

940 E. Baltimore Pk., Kennett Sq. (610) 388-1144 (in Chester Cty.)

This Italian-American is in Kennett Square, the heart of mushroom country, and though its appearance may be "rough and tumble," people go for the "great mushroom specialties." It's a "fun place," but voters say that beyond the fungi, the food is forgettable. A few say it's worse than that, and some complain of "appallingly rude" service.

 = Superior = Excellent = Very Good

Hunan Village

$18

1431 Old York Rd., Abington Shopping Center, Abington (215) 886-1229 (in Montgomery County)

It may only be one restaurant, but it has a village full of fans in Abington. This neighborhood Chinese, "a cut above your standard Chinese restaurant," may be located in the Abington Shopping Center, but is still "a favorite" to many hunanophiles. Suburban Chinese won't make it onto the national food registry, but if you're in the nabe, BYO and give it a shot. P.S. We made up the word "hunanophiles."

Hymie's Merion Deli

$13

342 Montgomery Ave., Merion (610) 668-DELI at Old Lancaster Rd. on the Main Line

Comments and votes are all over the map for this New York-style Deli in Merion, due partly to the huge response, and partly, we think, due to the reputation Hymie's has earned. It has everything a deli should, from "good bagels," "great breakfasts," and the "biggest sandwiches in the area," plus "classic" (read "rude") waitresses. "Where else can you see fur coats in a deli?"

Il Giardino

$27

Rt. 30 & Church Rd., Ardmore (610) 896-0705 on the Main Line

This Main Line Italian gets only average grades, especially from middle-aged voters who go most often. The New York-style atmosphere is dressy—jacket and tie are suggested—but the consensus is "OK, but there are better restaurants in the area."

Il Portico

VOTE

1519 Walnut St., Phila. (215) 587-7000 (bet. 15th & 16th in Ctr. City)

Finally—an Italian comes into the Walnut center of the Philadelphia dining scene. This formal Tuscan opened just after our survey was completed, but if the owners' other restaurant, Tira Misu, is any indication, Il Portico will be a winner.

Il Sol D'Italia

$34

255 N. Sycamore St., Newtown (215) 968-5880 (in Bucks Cty.)

To many voters, this "Italian sun," serving "very good" Southern Italian in Bucks County is truly the center of the universe. Simply put, "the food is fantastic," and by most accounts "underrated," and the menu is "imaginative." It's also a night spot: Wednesday, Friday and Saturday nights you'll find "good dancing and bands." If you are not young at heart, be warned: "Singles gather here."

Imperial Inn

$19

10th & Race Sts., Phila. (215) 627-2299, 627-5588 in Chinatown

While the ratings for this Chinatown standby don't exactly put it at the top of any lists, you'd never know it from the way our reviewers talk about it. Comments range from "very good" to the "best in Chinatown" (at least for the dim sum), to—and we think this must be big—"venerable." Here's a tip from one Sinophile: "It's even more authentic when you order from their Chinese language menu."

FOOD ROOM STAFF COST

Ingleneuk Tea House $20

120 Park Ave., Swarthmore (610) 543-4569 (in Delaware Cty.)

Afternoon tea is a thing of the past, even at this Swarthmore American, quite the same as since it opened 80 years ago. Some voters dismiss the old-fashioned menu and early American decor, saying it's "a good place to take your mother or grandmother, and that's about it." But if you appreciate "real homestyle food" with everything made from scratch ("try the fritters," voters say, and sticky buns are special), all dished up family-style by veteran waitresses, this is your place.

Inn Flight $23

1301 Old York Rd., Abington (215) 343-9967(Montgomery Cty.)
334 Easton Rd., Warrington (215) 343-9967 (Bucks County)
284 E. St., Feasterville/Trevose (215) 357-9988 (Bucks County)
2328 E. Lincoln Hwy., Langhorne (215) 752-5100 (Bucks County)
Rt. 309, Lansdale (215) 822-6610 (Bucks County)

The name of this Steak and Seafood chain begs for a comparison to airline food, but the "dark and smoky bar" atmosphere (that often "detracts from food enjoyment") makes that impossible since smoking was banned from all domestic flights. And, though the numbers are only fair to middling, they do at least support the comment that the quality is "consistent," if not outstanding.

Inn Philadelphia, The $33

251 S. Camac St., Philadelphia (215) 732-8630
bet. 12th & 13th, Locust & Spruce in Center City

Last year's complete renovation of this historic, Federal period Classic and Nouvelle Continental has produced (or reproduced) a charming atmosphere. The main dining room rises two stories high, and there's a more modern room where local art hangs on the wall and the locals themselves hang around the bar. This place is close to a breakthrough—one voter says "it could be tops with some fine tuning"—with big portions of "very good food" served by an "attentive staff." "Go—because you deserve it."

International Poultry Co. $10

2186 County Line Rd., Marketplace, Huntingdon Valley
(215) 953-1000 (at Davisville Rd. in Montgomery County)

You can get chicken, 10 different ways, and turkey dishes at this new Huntingdon Valley spot, though none of those 10 ways seems to please our voters very much. The average price is low, yet voters think it's "too high for their meals," and that there are "more and better ways to make chicken." "Change the name—it sounds like a slaughterhouse."

Io e Tu $27

1514-20 S. 9th St., Philadelphia (215) 271-3906
bet. Tasker & Dickenson in So. Phila.

The name may be Italian for "me and you," but everyone else gives this South Philly regional Italian only average marks overall. The vote is decidedly split, with the younger crowd giving it higher marks, especially for the food that one voter calls "not your usual Italian fare—imaginative!" Note: "imaginative" isn't always "excellent."

Irish Pub

$16

1123 Walnut St., Philadelphia (215) 925-3311
12th & Walnut Sts. in Center City
2007 Walnut St., Phila. (215) 568-5603 (at 20th St. in Ctr. City)
The food's American at this Center City saloon, but otherwise, the name says it all. Choose from a "good selection" of "cold beer," in an "excellent bar atmosphere," but while you're "enjoying drinks with friends," you may want to sample the snacks and "pass on dinner."

Isaac Newton's

$21

18 S. State St., Newtown (215) 860-5100 (in Bucks County)
Newton's first law of ordering is to keep it simple at this American Bistro, that's a "great place for a beer or a burger," but doesn't exactly hit you over the head with other options. The breads and salads are good, too, particularly "great" Caesar's, and the "really cool" atmosphere creates long lines, to get a seat overlooking the center of Newton. Go fig-ure.

Italian Bistro

$22

2500 Welsh Rd., Philadelphia (215) 934-7700
Welsh Rd. & Roosevelt Blvd. in Northeast Phila.
3401 Walnut St., Philadelphia (215) 387-7900
at 34th St. in University City/W. Phila.
"Surprisingly good," writes one voter. Well, creativity would be a surprise from an Italian Bistro with this name. "A great place for all," meaning families, say reviewers, though they are more inclined to talk about this mini-chain's more exotic locations, like "in the Ocean Mall in Atlantic City." The "nice bar" has an above-average selection of wines by the glass, and the pastries are also recommended. No reservations taken.

Jack's Firehouse

$35

2130 Fairmont Ave., Philadelphia (215) 232-9000
at 22nd St. in the Art Museum Area
Few places polarize voters like this Art Museum area American Regional—some think it's hot stuff, others think chef-owner Jack McDavid is blowing smoke. The lacquered wood of an old firehouse and "good beer on tap" make for a "manly" ambiance. The Southern-influenced food and custom-grown ingredients can "broaden your gastronomical horizons"; the menu changes daily, and game specials are "truly an adventure." But many think Jack's is "overexposed and overrated," "the epitome of style over substance," and even some who like the cooking say the staff can be "downright surly."

Jake and Oliver's House of Brews

VOTE

22 S. 3rd St., Philadelphia (215) 627-4825
bet. Market & Walnut Sts. in the Historic Area
The owners turned their ex-club, Revival, into this casual restaurant, which opened after our survey was completed. There are 40 microbrews on tap, (none of them Jake & Oliver's own), brick oven pizza and pub grub on the menu, dancing and DJ's Wed.-Sat. The panoramic mural of a wheatfield, done John Ford-style (lots of sky) could make Dorothy admit there IS a place like home.

FOOD ROOM STAFF COST

Jake's

$40

4365 Main St., Philadelphia (215) 483-0444 in Manayunk/Roxborough
This pioneering Manayunk New American earned its place among the region's favorite restaurants with its "hip yet elegant" atmosphere, "creative, interesting food" and "fabulous desserts," all served to look "as good as the murals on the wall." It's small but popular, so some complain that "tables are too close together," and there are quibbles about portion sizes and wine prices. The consensus, though, is that this is "Manayunk's greatest."

Jamaican Jerk Hut

$13

1436 South St., Philadelphia (215) 545-8644
at 15th St. in the South St. Area
If you're used to Americanized Jamaican food, getting used to the very spicy spices from the Spice Islands might "take some time." However, it's well worth it for the Caribbean atmosphere, and good "fun food." From the lousy decor, our voters advise you "take it home and enjoy it with a cold one." P.S. The low staff rating isn't because they're jerks, it's because they're too laid-back.

J.B. Winberie

$19

8229 Germantown Ave., Chestnut Hill Hotel, Phila. (215) 247-6710
at Southampton in Chestnut Hill/Mt. Airy
1164 Valley Forge Rd. Wayne (610) 293-9333
across from Gateway Shopping Center in Chester County
These chain Americans are popular with students, because the food is "inexpensive," the atmosphere is "relaxed," the servers are "friendly," and some locations have outdoor dining. The ratings are low, but you know what to expect: "stick to burgers and salads."

Jean-Pierre's

$57

101 S. State St., Newtown (215) 968-6201 in Bucks County
Don't be late for Jean-Pierre and Joan Tardy's great French cuisine at this little country restaurant in Newtown. With the perfunctory rustic fireplaces, it's in an unusually old building, the 1747 Thornton House. But the "best French food" comes at a price, that some feel is "too expensive." We're willing to wager an $85 prix fixe dinner that it's well worth it.

Jeannine's Bistro

$35

10 S. Front St., Philadelphia (215) 925-2928
bet. Market & Chestnut Sts. in the Historic Area
Voters say this Old City Country French Bistro, the casual upstairs complement to La Truffe, serves "the best *cassoulet* in town" in a cozy and romantic atmosphere. The wine list is extensive—more than two dozen are sold by the glass—and reservations are essential on weekends, especially Fridays, when Jeannine sings.

 = Superior = Excellent = Very Good

Jefferson House

$36

2519 DeKalb Pk., Norristown (610) 275-3407
S. of Germantown Pk. in Montgomery County

Many voters agree that you "don't get service like this anywhere else," from a professional staff that is very knowledgeable of the huge wine list (over 700 vintages are available by request, with 275 on the list). The food gets mixed results, with the majority of votes in the "very good" range, but all agree that the setting is "elegant," with "beautiful gardens and dining rooms." A special occasion place that is also kid-friendly, you're in good hands at the Jefferson.

Jenny's

$35

Rt. 202 & Street Rd., Peddlar's Village, Lahaska (215) 794-4020 in Bucks County

A "nice place to visit," this is the upscale Continental entry among the eight restaurants in Peddler's Village, the Central Bucks tourist spot. Younger voters are more likely to be bowled over by the cherry wood and tiffany lamp ambiance; older voters give the food just above-average grades. Reservations are essential, particularly for weekend nights, when jazz and blues bands play, and for the dixieland Sunday brunch.

Jill's Vorspeise

$8

12th & Filbert Sts., Reading Terminal Market, Philadelphia (215) 925-5415 in Center City

If you are what you eat, then get "fresh and healthy" at this soup/salad/health food spot in the Reading Terminal Market. The "charming, friendly, and good-looking" staff shops for the ingredients right in the Terminal the same day, then prepares it and serves it to you. The very good food rating underscores comments like "absolutely the best healthy lunch in the Market."

Jim's Steaks

$9

400 South St., Phila. (215) 928-1911 at 4th St. in the South St. Area

Nothing stirs the passion of Philadelphians like cheesesteaks. Although this South Street landmark is No. 1 in our survey, a few claim "the place is on the decline." Most, however, find the chrome-deco decor and cafeteria-style service "an integral part of the South Street experience." Among the selling points: "the best steaks brought to you by the meanest servers," "a wide beer selection," and a second-floor dining room with a view of "the people parade."

Joe's

$48

7th & Laurel Sts., Reading (610) 373-6794 (in Berks County)

Owner-chef Jack Czarnecki and his wild-mushroom mecca have been featured in People magazine and on national TV, yet voters still pick it as one of the area's top Sleepers. The setting, a small, modest room way out in Reading, has a lot to do with it. Reviewers say it's "worth the drive" for the "unusual menu," featuring "excellent" wild mushrooms and exotic game meats.

FOOD ROOM STAFF COST

Joe's Peking Duck House $18

925 Race St., Phila. (215) 922-3277 bet. 9th & 10th in Chinatown
Would YOU buy a Peking Duck from a guy named Joe? Plenty of our reviewers have, and though they warn this dive is perhaps the "most disgusting looking restaurant" in Philly, the food here is simply divine. They recommend the "best Peking duck for two," and advise that it is "cash only—but you don't have to bring much!"

Johnny Mott's $29

Cedarbrook Hill Apts., Wyncote (215) 887-1263
Rt. 309 & Greenwood Ave. in Montgomery County
Reservations are essential at this "consistently good" Cheltenham Italian seafooder. Johnny Mott's draws a mostly older crowd that gives its wide range of seafood dishes average marks. Early bird specials keep the prices reasonable.

John's Village Market $9

676 Lancaster Ave., Berwyn (610) 251-9720 on the Main Line
1 Pennsylvania Ave., Wayne (610) 688-2633
behind the Wayne Train Station on the Main Line
While they also serve fresh pizza in this appropriately wedge-shaped sandwich shop by the Wayne train station, John's has won its great reputation for serving the "best hoagie on the Main Line." They make the roast beef hoagie an art form, crowned with killer horseradish. Voters also love their turkey hoagies.

Jonathon's Deli $13

130 S. 11th St., Phila. (215) 829-8101
bet. Walnut & Sansom in Center City
You find traditional New York deli favorites and authentic Middle Eastern fare at this Center City Kosher. One voter sums it up: "What could be wrong? A local Jewish organization gets catered here."

Jon's Bar & Grill $18

3rd & South Sts., Phila. (215) 592-1390 in the South St. Area
While there's always "great people-watching on South Street," this may be the pick of the places from which to do it. With average food, at "reasonable prices," they've got an inner court, that keeps you off the street and puts this place in the Top 10 for outdoor dining. Plus, the kitchen stays open until 1am.

Joseph Ambler Inn $38

1005 Horsham Rd., Montgomeryville (215) 362-7500
Stump & Upper State Rds. in Montgomery County
"A lovely country inn in the heart of suburbia," the Joseph Ambler keeps locals and travelers well satisfied with "inspired" Continental and American cuisine. Whatever your opinion of country inns, dial it up a notch in all categories to imagine this place, which does very well across the boards. In fact, the only negative comment we heard was that the food can be "uneven at times." This historic location is also recommended for wedding rehearsal dinners.

 = Superior = Excellent = Very Good

Joseph's Italian

$27

1915 E. Passyunk Ave., Philadelphia (215) 755-2770
bet. Broad & 13th, Mifflin & McKean in So. Phila.

This New Age Italian, large by South Philly standards, mixes the best of the old and the new—modern decor, Sinatra and Pavarotti music, and a very good menu—Joseph gives veal, seafood and pasta classics a "very creative" spin. Prices are reasonable, and scores for the "great staff" have improved.

Joy Tsin Lau

$18

1026 Race St , Philadelphia (215) 592-7226
at 11th St. in Chinatown

Many of our voters are attracted to a place where the first two words sound like "joy" and "sin." But the "great dim sum" is the real star of this authentic Chinatown spot. In the supporting role, the decor is "one of the nicest in Chinatown," though "the service doesn't live up to the looks or the menu."

Judy's Cafe

$25

3rd & Bainbridge Sts., Philadelphia (215) 928-1968
in the South St. Area

"Judy, Judy, Judy," intones one Cary Grant impersonator, in awe of the "very good" home-cooked American food at this busy, mid-priced Queen Village spot, now it its twentieth year. In addition to having more votes per available seat than any other place, Judy's makes it to the top of many Romac lists: It's in the Top 30 for Philly's favorites, on the Top 10 list for best salad, and was voted #1 for gay and lesbian patrons. "Colorful clientele makes their delicious food that much more entertaining," they say, and the "huge portions" from a frequently changing menu make it all the better.

Julie's

$17

680 Easton Rd., Horsham (215) 442-1965
at Maple Ave. in Montgomery County

While they may not be the finest in the book, the steaks at this large Horsham American are "bigger than your head." The average Romac staff head measuring between eight and ten inches across, and weighing close to twenty pounds, that makes this place a "great value." With nostalgic decor (old Coke signs and the like), the "big surprise" at this casual, family place is the "great Caesar's."

Justin's Carriage House (fka Jus Dale's)

$27

3911 Skippack Pk., Skippack (610) 584-5005
at Rt. 73 in Montgomery County

A big selection of wines by the glass, "relaxed and comfortable" historic setting and live bands on Thursdays tend to offset the so-so ratings this Skippack Steak and Seafooder earns for its food. Only five years old, they changed their name, and take an old-fashioned approach to running a restaurant: low-stress if you bring the kids, and low-stress if you choose to smoke.

FOOD ROOM STAFF COST

JW's Steakhouse at the Phila. Marriott

VOTE

1201 Market St., Phila. (215) 625-2900 at 12th St. in Center City

Not many Romac Reporters have wandered into the dining room of the new Philadelphia Marriott. Those who have love the "huge dishes" of pasta and steak and the airy room, flanked by the hotel atrium, outdoor balconies and a wall of windows overlooking the street.

Kabul

$20

106 Chestnut St., Philadelphia (215) 922-3676
bet. Front & 2nd in the Historic Area

For those of you who rarely travel east of Milan on the culinary map, this Center City Afghan is a "good place to try some new, interesting and very good food." They have what one calls the "best chicken kebab in the city," at very reasonable prices that include a BYOB policy. But even if you're an old hand at Near Eastern cuisine, the ratings tell us it is truly "Afghan at its best."

Kansas City Prime

$51

4417 Main St., Phila. (215) 482-3700 at Gay St. in Manayunk

Despite arguments over whether this "expensive" Manayunk yearling is "overpriced" or not, most of the voters give KC Prime top marks for food, and often refer to it as "the best steakhouse in Philadelphia." Very good, very expensive cuts of beef are cooked to order, culminating with Philly's only option for Japanese Kobe steak. The price war breaks off into the now-famous potato skirmish, with diners asking "what potato is worth $4?"

Karla's

$29

5 W. Mechanic St., New Hope (215) 862-2612 (at Main St. in Bucks Co.)

What brings diners to this International bistro in New Hope? Could be the food, rated as "good," with an eclectic bill of fare that changes often. Could be the cozy atmosphere, with acoustic live jazz Monday through Friday nights, and a mural by local artist William Seles. But its most unique feature has to be the late light breakfast, served Friday and Saturday nights until 4a.m.

Kathryn's Inn

$23

4990 State Rd., Drexel Hill (610) 623-6900 at Twp. Line Rd. in Del. Co.

Though some say it's a "nice family place," voters give just fair grades to this Drexel Hill Italian/American. The best reason to visit is to listen to the "piano player who plays all the old, familiar favorites— very enjoyable."

Katmandu

$23

415 N. Delaware Ave., Philadelphia (215) 629-7400
bet. Spring Garden & Callowhill Sts. on the Delaware Riverfront

The granddaddy of the Delaware Avenue club scene packs in the crowds April through October. The American Bistro menu gets fair grades for "inconsistent" food, but voters like the outdoor dining with a view of the Ben Franklin Bridge, and live rock bands that crank up nightly.

 = Superior = Excellent = Very Good

Kawabata

$25

2455 Grant Ave., Philadelphia (215) 969-8225
at Roosevelt Blvd. in Northeast Phila.
110 Chestnut St., Philadelphia (215) 928-9564
bet. Front & 2nd in the Historic Area

They have a "great deal on all-you-can-eat sushi" Monday through Wednesday at these Northeast Philly/Center City Japanese spots, and that seems to be the best time to go: comments, particularly about the freshness of the fish, range from "creative and fresh" to "fishy," so a day with high volume can't hurt. Most agree it's "friendly and fun" but that the staff may have a darker side, and what is "laid back" service to some is a staff that "needs training" to others.

Kelly's Seafood

$24

9362 Old Bustleton Ave., Philadelphia (215) 969-5950
Welsh Rd. & Bustleton Ave./Roosevelt Blvd. in Northeast Phila.

This father, sons and daughter establishment on Old Bustleton Avenue is proud to say they've always had a Kelly in the kitchen. This place feels like it's been here forever, and though that may mean the food needs a bit of sprucing up, it is still a comfortable choice.

Kennedy-Supplee Mansion

$41

Rt. 23 at Valley Forge Park, King of Prussia (610) 337-3777
in Montgomery County

While it's "too bad that the food doesn't match the room," the room is of very high quality. Located in Valley Forge Park, this historic house has been "beautifully maintained," overshadowing everything else. "A very romantic spot," you'll have to "reserve in advance for that special evening." Some say it's worth getting dressed up and driving to King of Prussia just to see the "large, lavish ladies' room." Priced at the high end.

Kimberton Inn

$34

Hares Hill & Kimberton Rds., Kimberton (610) 933-8148
in Chester County

Many rave, some yawn about the Continental food at this historic crossroads inn outside Phoenixville, but there's wide acclaim for the "pastoral, serene" upscale setting, highlighted by fresh flowers from the on-site gardens, piano and harp music, and an excellent staff. Coffee is a specialty.

King George II Inn

$35

102 Radcliffe St., Bristol (215) 788-5536
Mill & Radcliffe in Bucks County

This Bristol spot claims it is America's oldest operating inn, so naturally it has a "fairly traditional menu" of "delicious" American-Continental fare, and a large selection of wines by the glass to go with it. Its best scores, though, are for the atmosphere: "cozy, romantic" bar, piano music, and a "great view" of the Delaware—"make sure you sit downstairs by the window."

FOOD ROOM STAFF COST

King Street Grill

$12

5 W. King St., Malvern (610) 644-2644
on the Main Line

Many of our reviewers who are interested in heart-healthy food have been turning their attention to the light grills that have been springing up. This Eclectic American, specializing in breakfast and lunch in Malvern, has become one of the first picks, and an inexpensive one at that. It's "the best place to meet the locals" at "the best breakfast in PA!" At whatever meal, this place is packed.

Knave of Hearts

$27

230 South St., Philadelphia (215) 922-3956
bet. 2nd & 3rd Sts. in the South St. Area

Like the playing card, this South Street International and Eclectic restaurant seems to have two sides. While it has great, Top 10-rated salads, places very high in our popularity poll, and is a "romantic" "great date restaurant," many say the service could use more training, or at least cordiality lessons. "One decent visit, one so-so," is typical of our voters reactions, as is "one bartender's great—one's nasty!"

Knickers

$16

1650 Limekiln Pk., Dresher (215) 646-2856
in Montgomery County

This golf-themed, middle-of-the-fairway pub-style American/Continental in Dresher is popular with the locals, whether they're looking for a wide selection of beers or a spot to take the family for dinner. Voters applaud the recently opened bakery and say it's "especially fun for lunch." Call for reservations if you're more than a foursome.

La Bonne Auberge

$62

Village 2, off Mechanic St., New Hope (215) 862-2462
in Bucks County

One of New Hope's top entries in the Classic French category, La Bonne Auberge is situated in a restored, pre-revolutionary war farmhouse and has won many fans, who dress up for "very romantic," if "expensive" meals. "A very special place," though the food is sometimes "inconsistent," there are certain things you should expect going in: reserve, dress up, and note the "three-figure wine prices."

La Buca

$39

711 Locust St., Philadelphia (215) 928-0556
bet. 7th & 8th in the Historic Area

If there is some disagreement over the food, it is between "very good" and "excellent" at this Tuscan restaurant in the Historic Area. Though the name of the place may mean "the goat," the emphasis is on fish, with perhaps "the best Dover sole" as a standout. There's a "nice selection of wines" and "good atmosphere," and the staff also wins raves.

 = Superior = Excellent = Very Good

La Campagna

60 E. Baltimore Pk., Clifton Heights (610) 626-6036
at Diamond St. in Delaware County

Chef/owner Daniel Lewis and wife Carolyn create a cordial atmosphere at this Clifton Heights Italian that some reviewers call "close to home." But all that friendliness doesn't mean you won't get one of the best Italian meals west of South Philly. "A fine place to go," for "good" food, pretty decor and weekend entertainment.

La Cocotte

$34

124 W. Gay St., West Chester (610) 436-6722
Church & Darlington Sts. in Chester County

Romac Reporters visit this downtown West Chester spot for "classic French at reasonable prices." The menu changes seasonally. A few rate the room and staff as so-so; others say it's a "great place for a romantic dinner."

La Collina

$45

37-41 Ashland Ave., Belmont Hills (610) 668-1780 on the Main Line

The ratings have picked up at this near-Manayunk Main Liner, which serves "very good" Northern Italian food in a "classy," jacket-and-tie-required atmosphere. In the midst of all this elegance, some of the many diners who have visited this place feel slighted, whether for "waiting despite reservations," or because they think it's "too pricey." Maybe just didn't get a table by the window, with a view of the Schuykill, or by one of the four fireplaces. Dress up, and remember your dancing shoes.

La Famiglia

$47

8 S. Front St., Philadelphia (215) 922-2803
bet. Market & Chestnut Sts. in the Historic Area

This Old City spot is "the best Italian restaurant in Philadelphia" for many voters, who love its "fresh fish" and "light yet rich northern Italian" cuisine. They also like the "elegant and intimate" atmosphere and the selection of 900 wines, nearly all from Italy. Some love the European service, though a few think it's "snobby," and there's widespread grumbling about the prices.

La Fourchette

$46

110 N. Wayne Ave., Wayne (610) 687-8333 at Lancaster Ave. on the Main Line

The "sterling" reputation of The Fork is well deserved, with high marks "all around," especially for its attentive service. "The food is superbly presented, and exceptionally delicious," says one satisfied customer, "the best on the Main Line," adds another. While elegant, the ambiance has a split personality—upstairs it is more formal, for quiet, special occasions, but downstairs it is a touch more casual and is good for people-watching. After recent criticism, the food portions have increased, without sacrificing quality—"we felt privileged," says one couple, the appropriate way to rave like a Main Liner.

FOOD ROOM STAFF COST

La Fourno

$14

636 South St., Phila. (215) 627-9000 at 7th St. in the South St. Area
Many think the wood-burning brick oven at this South Street pizzeria turns out the "best pizza in Philly," especially the veggie pies, but that's not the only reason many chose this as a sleeper worth mentioning. The pasta dishes and *panini* (Italian sandwiches) are also popular, which is why the kitchen is expanding the menu.

Lagoon

$19

101 Taylor Ave., Essington (610) 521-1400 at Rt. 420 S. in Del. Co.
This Essington nightspot overlooks the Delaware River and, like Philly's river clubs, is entertainment-oriented. Voters say the kitchen serves "typical bar food," but the place has a "great view" and feels "like a day at the shore." The crowd? "Bring your hairspray."

La Grolla

$33

782 S. 2nd St., Philadelphia (215) 627-7701
bet. Fitzwater & Catherine Sts. in So. Phila.
Here's one Italian that keeps alive the tradition of great South Philly restaurants. Serving "true Northern Italian" food, in a "homey" if unspectacular setting, the service is impeccable, and the specials truly earn that moniker: with the "best Carpaccio in town," they also serve an "amazing wild game dinner," 15 courses, at a fixed price of under $60. Call ahead and see what other feasts are planned.

Lake House Inn

$37

1100 Old Bethlehem Rd., Perkasie (215) 257-5351
Elephant & Three Mile Run Rds. in Bucks County
An historic setting gives the six dining rooms, with lovely views of Lake Nockamixon, a charming, New England Inn feeling. In spite of a professional staff and reasonable prices, this food only pulls down average ratings. Kid-friendly, there's a good Sunday brunch, early bird specials, and a fair selection of wines by the glass. Closed Mondays.

Landing

$34

22 N. Main St., New Hope (215) 862-5711 in Bucks County
Appropriated named, since the food, though often "delicious," is also "expensive," and thus far hasn't taken off. In nice weather, the capacity of this Delaware Riverside Contemporary American triples: While it is like grandmother's house inside, the place to be is on the porch, enjoying "beautiful" views. A "pleasant place to relax on a nice summer evening."

La Padella

$30

1619 Grant Ave., Grant Plaza II, Philadelphia (215) 677-7723
bet. Bustleton Ave. & Kreuztown Rd. in Northeast Phila.
Nestled in the Grant Avenue Shopping Center, it's not much to look at from the outside, but that "does not represent the food or atmosphere inside." Voters call it a "real sleeper in the Northeast—good, with a great piano bar." In all, it does well for a strip mall restaurant that diners could have panned.

 = Superior = Excellent = Very Good

La Paella Tio Pepe

$27

12012 Bustleton Ave., Philadelphia (215) 677-8016
bet. Byberry Rd. & Hendrix St. in Northeast Phila.

With his co-owner and wife Conchita standing by, Uncle Pepe is in the kitchen cooking up "homestyle" Spanish dishes, with some French and Portuguese specialties in the mix. It is cozy inside, with arched doorways and other Spanish touches. Ingredients come fresh from the chef's garden, so the food can be a "great treat." "Go for the early bird special," and try the homemade sangria.

La Scala's Copper Penny

$24

237 St. James Pl., Phila. (215) 925-1802
2nd & Dock Sts. in the Historic Area

A penny for Romac Reporters' thoughts seems like a fair return on this Society Hill Italian-American, which won't win any gold medals—or even bronze. The wide-ranging menu, reasonable prices, cozy room and Sinatra music might make it in South Philly, but people in this part of town seem to have higher expectations.

Last Drop Coffeehouse

$8

13th & Pine Sts., Philadelphia (215) 893-0434
in Center City

One of the top-ranked coffeehouses in Philly, it comes from the old school: with local artists on the walls, and local musicians off the walls, it's a "hangout for alternatives, with punkers playing chess." "Smoky," you can try and block some of those free-radicals at the just-opened juice bar. "It's a dive, but a great dive, and"—oh yeah—"great coffee."

La Truffe

$49

10 S. Front St., Philadelphia (215) 925-5062
at Market St. in the Historic Area

Though not exactly buried, this charming Contemporary French dining room is like its namesake, the truffle, in many ways. For starters, the food is exquisite, earning an "excellent" rating, a top 30 ranking, and comments like "top shelf" and "a legacy." It's also romantic, with a "beautiful dining room" and a top-notch staff. One diner says it's "like Le Bec-Fin but much more comfortable." The prix fixe, though expensive, is a delightful introduction to the many facets of the truffle.

La Veranda

$41

Pier 3, Penns Landing, Philadelphia (215) 351-1898
bet. Market & Arch on the Delaware Riverfront

The view of the Delaware from the two-floor patio at this Penn's Landing Italian is among the top on the survey, but it doesn't overshadow the strong food ratings. Voters cry "magnifico!" for the authentic antipasto table, "great grilled vegetables" and "very fresh fish selections." The service receives very good marks—while a few voters grumble, most feel "pampered."

FOOD ROOM STAFF COST

La Vigna

$32

1100 S. Front St., Philadelphia (215) 336-1100
at Federal St. in So. Phila.

It means "the vine," and according to many of our voters, particularly the younger set, the food is divine to match, with the staff running a close second. With a renovation that is due to be completed at the publication of this book, this South Philly Northern Italian "old pals' hangout" has a lot going for it. Poke your head in the private dining room on your way out.

Le Bar Lyonnais

$41

1523 Walnut St., Philadelphia (215) 567-1000
bet. 15th & 16th in Center City

This Center City French bistro, the downstairs offspring of Le Bec-Fin, has "superb everything," including some of the best bar food in the city, like "mashed potatoes to die for." Many say the "great romantic atmosphere" makes it a natural for dessert and champagne before or after the theater. Reservations not taken.

Le Bec-Fin

$99

1523 Walnut St., Philadelphia (215) 567-1000
bet. 15th & 16th in Center City

"How many superlatives are left?" wonders one Romac Reporter about chef/owner Georges Perrier's internationally acclaimed Center City French restaurant, No. 1 on our survey for food. Meals are prix fixe, wine not included—"lunch is a bargain" at $32. Dinner is "worth every cent" at $97, and is served in several courses, including cheese and dessert. The rooms are "elegant," the staff is "excellent," though some complain that "service at lunch is getting too mechanical." Reserve weeks in advance for an "event," a "a total experience."

Le Bus Main St.

$19

4266 Main St., Philadelphia (215) 487-2663
bet. Cotton & Rector in Manayunk/Roxborough

For "good" American food in Manayunk, and the top baked goods on our survey, make a Le Bus Stop. The homemade bread is "awesome," and while the menu strikes younger voters as "simple and inventive," the middle-aged are more likely to find it "dull." It's fun for kids, thanks to a toy box in the waiting area (you'll need it—reservations are limited to parties of six or more), but service sometimes wilts under the crowds. One common complaint—"if Le Bus weren't so popular," one voter says, "maybe the staff would be nicer to you."

Le Bus Sansom St.

$13

3402 Sansom St., Philadelphia (215) 387-3800
at 34th St. in University City/W. Phila.

The crowds pack David Braverman's cafeteria-style American restaurant, that also supplies the breads for many other local spots. "Terrific coffee, breads and pastries" are just the beginning, with "the best tuna fish" among the other good choices. For a less "utilitarian" atmosphere, try the table service Manayunk location.

Le Champignon

$43

122 Lombard St., Philadelphia (215) 922-2515
bet. Front & 2nd Sts. in the Historic Area

This Society Hill restaurant's unique combination of Japanese, French and Thai cooking lets you start a meal with sushi or escargots, in either a classic French dining room or a traditional tatami room. Early bird specials and prix fixe dinners help keep the tab within reason. Service receives very good marks, and a few say "everything is delicious" on the "schizophrenic menu," but others want to know, "How did this great restaurant go downhill?"

Lee How Fook

$15

219 N. 11th St., Philadelphia (215) 925-7266
in Chinatown

While this teeny Chinatown Cantonese may well win the prize for worst room and ambiance ("absolutely no atmosphere," claims one reviewer) it has very good food, with "great salt-baked squid" and excellent hot-and-sour soups as standouts. With other specialties like "shrimp on hot rock salt," when you're bringing your own wine or beer, we suggest you bring along a jug of water, too.

Lee's Hoagies

$10

4034 Walnut St., Philadelphia (215) 387-0905
bet. 40th & 41st in University City & many other locations

Like many local chains, votes vary with the quality of the nearest shop. Some rave it's "the best hoagie in America," with "huge sandwiches that are a great value." Others say they're "overpriced, and the quality is not high." One unique feature is the "traveling hoagie," with the innards wrapped in wax paper to prevent the roll from turning soggy.

Lemon Grass Thai

$22

3630 Lancaster Ave., Philadelphia (215) 222-8042
1 Blk. N. of Market in University City/W. Phila.

"The menu is x-rated, but the food is superb" at this University City Thai. No, they're not referring to the pictures of the meals, but the names, like "Evil Jungle Princess," "Sweet Surrender," "Screaming Mermaid," and "Young Girl on Fire." Lemon Grass also has an extensive vegetarian menu. With "great staff and service," low budget Penn and Drexel students say "the prices could be better."

Lenape Inn

$30

1333 Lenape Rd., West Chester (610) 793-2005 in Chester County

How's this for the dream date: "very good food," in a "quiet and romantic" setting, with enough seats that, no matter how busy they are, you won't be waiting long at the bar. Cap it off with a "wall of windows" that offers very "pretty views of the Brandywine River," two fireplaces, and a professional, courteous staff, and you have the makings for one of the great dates of all time.

= Good = Fair [no rating] = Poor

FOOD ROOM STAFF COST

Le Petit Cafe

$34

7026 Terminal Sq., Upper Darby (610) 352-8040
69th & Market Sts. in Delaware County

Why can't France and Northern Italy just get along? They do, very nicely at this little spot in Terminal Square in Upper Darby. The French country look is complemented by great grilled meat dishes, including rack of lamb and "the best duck." With lighter options available, it's "perfect for a quiet evening," and is a real crowd, uh, little crowd pleaser. BYO.

Liberties

$26

705 N. 2nd St., Philadelphia (215) 238-0660
at Fairmount Ave. in Northern Liberties

This antique-filled Victorian bistro in Northern Liberties features Modern American food with a French influence that Romac Reporters, especially younger ones, call "really good." The prices are reasonable, the room has character (hand-carved mahogany bar, tin ceilings, you know the drill), and voters "always feel welcome here—it's not pretentious at all." Swing by on a weekend for the live jazz combos.

Lickety Split

$24

401 South St., Philadelphia (215) 922-1173
4th & South Sts. in the South St. Area

Sometimes a carefully worded evaluation by a voter can speak volumes about a restaurant. Often, simple praise of a special dish is all we need to get a handle on a place. But in the case of this South Street joint, serving burgers, pasta and simple seafood dishes, and with a bar that is twice as big as the dining room, one anecdote tells it all: "I got really drunk here."

Lily Langtry's at the Sheraton Valley Forge

$36

1160 First Ave., King of Prussia (610) 337-5459
at 363 N. in Montgomery County

Dinner theater is, well, alive at this hotel restaurant out in a lovely country setting near Valley Forge. While the "entertainment is good," including a Las Vegas-style revue, our voters can't say as much for the food. Still, the very curious will love it for the nostalgic decor, and big groups can buy the place out for the evening. Reserve ahead for the timed seatings.

Little Inn

$23

9 State Rd., Media (610) 565-8212 at Rt. 252 in Delaware County

With its Continental menu, quaint Victorian decor, weekday early bird specials for seniors and weekend piano background music, this spot in the heart of Media, "good for many years," seems aimed at an older audience. But it gets higher marks and more traffic from younger voters, who find "good American cooking and great crab cakes," along with "good people watching."

 = Superior = Excellent = Very Good

Little Pete's

$12

219 S. 17th St., Philadelphia (215) 545-5508
17th & Chancellor Sts. in Center City
19th & Chestnut Sts., Philadelphia (215) 563-2303 in Center City
2400 Fairmount Ave., Philadelphia (215) 232-5001 at 24th St. in the Art Museum Area

A dumpy room and low food and staff ratings don't matter to the large crowd who frequent these diners. Reubens and cheesesteaks receive praise, though in the same, coughing breath our voters warn that the rooms can get smoky. "Great if you want a cheap meal at any hour."

Logan Inn

$28

10 W. Ferry St., New Hope (215) 862-2300
S. Main & Ferry in Bucks County

A primarily over-30 crowd tells us Logan's runs with an average staff in an average, if historic atmosphere. The American food, however, isn't up to that of the other New Hope country inns, though it is available on two menus: the "fine dining" menu, with pasta, chicken, filet and the like, and the simpler, standby cafe menu. Breakfast is a standout.

Log Cabin

VOTE

11 Lehoy Forest Dr., Leola (717) 626-1181
6 miles north of Lancaster off Rt. 272 in Lancaster County

Don't let the name fool you. This Lancaster County spot was born as a log cabin, but renovations have made it one of the area's fanciest, priciest and most praised dining spots. The room is decorated with fine art; the locals say the steaks are the best bet on the American/Continental menu.

London Grill

$28

2301 Fairmount Ave., Philadelphia (215) 978-4545
at 23rd St. in the Art Museum Area

Though the dining room gets good grades, the "great bar food and happy hour" distinguish this very popular Art Museum area New American. The menu's "unique choices" are "interesting and well thought out," even if the "service is sporadic." But all agree "the bar is a special place, friendly and laid-back," a "neat place to hang out"—especially from 5 to 7 p.m., every day but Saturday, when the bar menu is half-price.

Long's Gourmet Chinese

$19

2018 Hamilton St., Philadelphia (215) 496-9928
bet. 20th & 21st Sts. in the Art Museum Area

It's probably the Art Museum Area location that makes this little restaurant so expensive for Chinese. According to our Romac Reporters, it is not the quality of the food. Long's contemporary menu includes classic Szechuan and Cantonese items, with special diet dishes, even Kosher dishes during passover. "Quiet and elegant," doesn't make up for "overpriced Chinese" that's "really not that good."

FOOD ROOM STAFF COST

Longwood Inn

$27

Rt. 1, Kennett Square (610) 444-3515 at Rt. 52 in Chester County
Don't let the "bad entrance" to this Kennett Square American keep you away, "if you're at the Gardens, it's simply a must!" While the prices are average, the "great crabcakes" and "quite good service" mark this spot as a "good value," especially when it comes to the Friday night seafood buffet. Homemade desserts complete the picture.

Lucky Star

$16

8919 Ridge Ave., Philadelphia (215) 482-3760 in Roxborough
"The food keeps getting better," even if the "staff needs to learn more English." Well, it doesn't make them any less "friendly," or hurt their rating, but adds to the authenticity of this Roxborough Chinese. "They make you feel at home," that is, if the decor in your home is "fair," and somebody cooks "good" Chinese food there. They have a small wine selection, and our voters recommend the takeout.

Maccabeam

$14

128 S. 12th St., Phila. (215) 922-5922 at Sansom St. in Center City
Read into the ratings, and you have a pretty good idea of what this Middle Eastern/Kosher/Israeli spot in Center City is like: good food ("best Middle East" to a few voters), with a lackluster room and so-so service in a kid-friendly environment. While you "can't beat it for hummus and tahini," one Romac Reporter put it this way: "authentic kosher food, indifferent staff, screaming kids."

Mace's Crossing

$15

1714 Cherry St., Phila. (215) 564-5203 17th & Pkwy. in Center City
This Center City bar is a popular watering hole in a 19th-century carriage house, but voters turn thumbs down on the low-priced, "mediocre" American Pub fare and a "staff full of bad attitude." "Mace the place."

Magnolia Cafe

$24

16th & Locust Sts., Philadelphia (215) 546-4180
A very large number of voters recommend this Cajun/Creole spot, with good "atmosphere and food to match." Not just another historic double brownstone in Center City, one voter calls it "old-faithful: always reliable, always nice, always there." With few Cajuns to pick from in Philly, Magnolia does a good job representing the bayou, serving "hot gumbo to a cool crowd." A minority of voters complain about the place, especially where service is concerned.

Main-ly Desserts

$14

4247 Main St., Phila. (215) 487-1325 at Rector St. in Manayunk
You've just had a great meal in Manayunk, but could use a little digestion time before dessert. Why not leave the restaurant and walk to Anne Gallagher's place? Chef John Vliet creates some of our voters' favorite desserts, including "mile high chocolate pie" and the "best strawberry shortcake in the universe," served with "great" coffee. It's "mainly yummy but mostly pricey for a regular stopover."

 = Superior = Excellent = Very Good

Mainland Inn

$40

17 Main St., Mainland (215) 256-8500 in Montgomery County

Romac Reporters call this quiet 1890 Montgomery County inn "a great find" and "an ultimate experience" that's "still something of a secret." The creative American cuisine, "made with the freshest ingredients" and artfully presented, is served in "rather formal" setting—jackets and ties are a good idea, and reservations are a must. "A first-class staff" and "attention to detail" add up to an experience "too fine for words."

Mama's Pizzeria

$11

426 Belmont Ave., Bala Cynwyd (610) 664-4757
at Levering Mill Rd. on the Main Line

This Main Line spot has pizza in its name, but it's the cheesesteaks that win Romac Reporters' hearts: They're slow-cooked, "overflowing with cheese" and "leave Pat's and Geno's in the dust." In winter, Mama's will freeze them and express-mail them anywhere in the country. In summer, far-flung fans have to "come home to Mama's!"

Ma Ma Yolanda's

$25

746 S. 8th St., Philadelphia (215) 592-0195
bet. Fitzwater & Catherine in So. Phila.

Antiques and marble statues distinguish the decor at this South Philly restaurant. Despite the Northern Italian menu, voters say "South Philly is spoken here." While not as low as some local red-gravy restaurants, prices are reasonable.

Mamma Maria's

$36

1637 E. Passyunk Ave., Philadelphia (215) 463-6884
bet. Morris & Tasker, 11th & 12th in So. Phila.

This South Philly Italian serves prix fixe menus: $13 for a three-course lunch, $35 for a seven-course dinner. Modest wine is included, but you can also bring your own. The Abruzzese food gets variable grades and the room is plain, but the very good service and accordian player on Saturday nights add up to old-world appeal.

Mandarin Garden

$18

1736 Chestnut St., Phila. (215) 567-1059 at 18th St. in Center City

They've kept the decor simple at this Center City Chinese, which seems to fit the reliable, if standard Mandarin, Szechuan and Cantonese food here. It's what you might expect: standard pricing, with tasty "hot and sour and seaweed soups" and a BYO policy. Think of it as a departure from your normal lunch routine.

Mandarin Garden

$21

91 N. York Rd., Willow Grove (215) 657-3993
at Davisville Rd. in Montgomery County

This Willow Grove Chinese might not look like much, but Romac Reporters give high praise to the "good, consistent" food, especially the "excellent Szechuan" dishes. With dim sum and a $19.95 prix fixe dinner, there's something for everyone. One voter even says it's "the only Chinese food I'll eat!"

FOOD ROOM STAFF COST

Manny Brown's

$17

512 South St., Philadelphia (215) 627-7427
bet. 5th & 6th in the South St. Area

Voters are blunt about this South Street Tex-Mex: It's a handy place to munch on big portions of fair Southwestern fare, but the toughest decision is what you'll wash it down with—there are 14 beers on tap, nearly 50 more in bottles.

Marabella's

$22

602 Skippack Pk., Blue Bell (215) 641-9100 in Montgomery Co.
1420 Locust St., Phila. (215) 545-1845 bet. 14th & 15th
17th & Ben Franlin Pkway., Phila. (215) 981-5555 in Center City
401 City Ave., Bala Cynwyd (610) 668-5353 in the City Line Area

From Center City to Blue Bell, "swinging singles" have a "loud and dark" place to go. Though the rooms may "echo," the food is generally "good," the staff "pleasant," and the ambiance, well, seems to be what you make it. But don't count the food out yet, they "grill foods well," they have "interesting vegetable combinations," and a new executive chef should improve the rest of the menu.

Marathon Grill

$12

16th & Sansom Sts., Philadelphia (215) 569-3278 in Center City
Suburban Station, Philadelphia (215) 564-4745 in Center City
1818 Market St., Philadelphia (215) 561-1818
bet. 18th & 19th in Center City

Though the Market Street location features a live-jazz happy hour, most Romac Reporters still view the Marathon as the quintessential quick-lunch place—fast, clean and healthy. "Fresh salads" are the big draw—tuna pasta and Caesar chicken win high praise. Dissenters say it's "overpriced" and decry the "yuppie festival" atmosphere.

Marbles

$18

818 Lancaster Ave., Bryn Mawr (610) 520-9100
next to the Bryn Mawr movie theater on the Main Line

Many of our voters yell about Marbles, partly due to the good American Bistro food with Middle Eastern influences, but mostly because they are temporarily deafened by the "unbearable noise level." "Cute waitresses, but bad acoustics," bellows one diner, but despite the decibel level and "tables crowded together," most admit they "love the food," that's also a "good value."

Margaret Kuo's Mandarin

$18

190 Lancaster Ave., Malvern (610) 647-5488
at Malin Rd. on the Main Line

The "nice decor" (referred to by the owners as "Miami Vice Oriental") is the first thing that hits you at this Malvern Chinese restaurant. But the "consistently good food," that may well be the "best in the Western Suburbs" will stay with you. The delicious seasoning will stay on your mind, while the large portions, "fairly priced," are usually enough to supply you with a doggy bag.

Margarita's

$18

200 Spring Ln., West Chester (610) 696-9720
Rt. 30 & W. Chester Pk. in Chester County

This West Chester Southwestern gets ho-hum grades for food and service—it's more the room, and the dancing and entertainment on weekends, that interest reviewers, especially the younger ones who rate it most kindly.

Marita's Cantina

$17

424 Bethlehem Pk., Fort Washington (215) 646-0867
in Montgomery County
610 E. Lancaster Ave., Bryn Mawr (610) 527-8989
on the Main Line

These suburban Mexicans received just fair ratings, yet they don't lack for customers. "Marita's is a great place for a quick drink with friends," "or for the lunchtime buffet," or to "celebrate Cinqo de Mayo." A few say "daily specials have been refreshingly tasty," but more describe it as "OK" and "so-so" and say, "If you're used to the good stuff, this place won't thrill you."

Marker at the Adams Mark Hotel

$38

City Ave. & Monument Rd., Philadelphia (215) 581-5010
Rt. 1 & Schuylkill Expy. in the City Line Area

Since we reported this "top notch but seemingly unknown" City Line restaurant as a sleeper last year, the number of voters has increased dramatically, and the results are simply superb. Executive chef Vincent Alberici uses only the freshest organic ingredients in his New American (with some European, and even Asian influences) dishes. While the view could improve, diners are satisfied to look inside the restaurant, at the split-level, antique-appointed dining room. The staff is utterly professional at this dressy spot, well worth getting past the "commercial look" of the hotel lobby. Brunch is a standout.

Marrakesh

$29

517 S. Leithgow St., Philadelphia (215) 925-5929
bet. 4th & 5th, South & Lombard Sts. in the South St. Area

"If you want to make a real experience of your meal, and feel like you're in another land, go" to this "authentic and fun" Moroccan in the South Street area. The food is good, and everyone loves the room and the staff. The price is "reasonable," especially when you consider the $20, 7-course prix fixe. It's "Morocco without the airfare."

Marra's

$18

1734 E. Passyunk Ave., Philadelphia (215) 463-9249 in So. Phila.

This "South Philly tradition" specializes in "great pizza"—pickier reviewers say "skip the rest of the food." Marra's brick oven is older than most restaurants in the city—it and the D'Adamo family have been giving patrons "the true ethnic feel of South Philly" since 1927. It's a popular stop for sports fans heading for a game, and voters say "for what it is, it can't be beat."

= Good = Fair [no rating] = Poor

FOOD ROOM STAFF COST

Marrone's Cafe

$14

2744 E. County Line Rd., Ardmore (610) 642-9567
bet. Ardmore Ave. & Wynnewood Rd. on the Main Line

The "pizza with triple cheese is a must" at this neighborhood Italian restaurant in Ardmore, now in its fiftieth year. And it's not just the locals that are drawn to the good food, especially the lobster ravioli: "I drove one hour to eat here," says one reviewer, "for quality that has been the same for the past 25 years."

Marshalton Inn

$35

1300 W. Strasburg Rd., West Chester (610) 692-4367
in Chester County

Diners have been able to get a meal at this Chester County Continental since Colonial furniture was considered modern. Nowadays people go for the "very authentic, sparse" candlelit decor—"it's like visiting life in the 1800's"—and, in the summer, for live entertainment on the outdoor deck. The food gets solid if unspectacular grades.

Martine's

VOTE

7 E. Ferry St., New Hope (215) 862-2966
Main St. across from the cannon in Bucks County

If you're in a romantic mood, "insist that you get seated upstairs" at this New Hope Northern Italian. Downstairs, you find what feels like an English Pub, with the bar as the centerpiece, while upstairs the room looks more like a French Bistro. Despite the two levels, the place is very small, and triples in capacity when outside dining is available. And, the food is "very good," the atmosphere "wonderful," though some feel the "staff gives the impression that it could not care less" about the customers.

Martini's

$16

852 Lancaster Ave., Devon (610) 688-9343
at Berkley Rd. on the Main Line

This Devon family Italian has been a favorite with the horse show crowd for decades. Voters flock here for old-fashioned pasta favorites, especially "delicious ravioli." With so many considering this the "best value sit-down Italian on the Main Line" (with the emphasis on value) and with a no-reservations policy, "be prepared to wait." No credit cards.

Mary's

$22

400 Roxborough Ave., Philadelphia (215) 487-2249
at Pechin St. in Manayunk/Roxborough

This tiny Manayunk BYO, the No. 1 favorite Vegetarian in the survey, packs them in for "the best veggie food"—"so creative." It has to be—no dairy products or sugar are used, though the kitchen does serve fish. Fans say you can "expect to wait 30-45 minutes from the time you place your order, but it's well worth it!" Brunch is popular: Featured are pancakes, waffles and crepes, all made with fresh-ground flour.

 = Superior **= Excellent** **= Very Good**

Mayfair Diner

$14

7373 Frankford Ave., Phila. (215) 624-8886 at Bleigh St. in NE Phila.

This steel-sided American classic in the Northeast is Philly's "closest thing to a Jersey diner—and that's a compliment!" For the uninitiated, that means it's "clean," serves "basic, mom-style food" (crab cakes are noteworthy) and a few feel its "waitresses need an attitude adjustment." Open 24 hours.

McCloskey's Bar

$15

17 Cricket Ave., Ardmore (610) 642-9280 at Rt. 30 on the Main Line

A wee bit o' the new transformed this Irish pub in Ardmore from a dingy taproom to a decent burger-and-beer spot. The simple, inexpensive food (reviewers recommend the mushroom soup) draws a mixed crowd, including parents with kids, early in the evening. After 10, younger folk come in to graze the pub menu.

McCrossen's Tavern

529 N. 20th St., Phila. (215) 854-0923 in the Art Museum Area

While the food is Continental with a Mediterranean flair, you will find everything here you'd expect at a good tavern. Unassuming menu items combine with the historic, exposed brick-and-mahogany setting to produce a "comfy neighborhood bar." The highest compliment for such a place: it's "the best hangout." Low prices mean you don't have to shell out, either.

McGillin's Olde Ale House

$16

1310 Drury Ln., Phila. (215) 735-5562 bet. 13th & Juniper in Center City

"A great setting with history" sums up the oldest tavern in Philadelphia. Opened 135 years ago, it has a wide selection of draft beers, and the place is actually pretty large for one so old. While the pub food is only fair, you can supplement your calorie intake with a pint of Guiness, though one reviewer complains "no draft Guinness upstairs."

Mediterraneo

$32

303 Horsham Rd., Horsham (215) 672-5595 at Rt. 611 in Mont. Co.

If you want very good food, or just want to brush up on your Italian with the friendly waiters from the old country, drop by owner Salvatore Carratta's Regional Italian restaurant in Horsham. We hear they have a "very good antipasto table," good wines by the glass, and a piano bar from Wednesday to Saturday. Reserveo in advanceo for weekend nights.

Medora's Mecca

$27

13th St. & Packer Ave., Phila. (215) 336-1655 in So. Phila.

Good food, and a mix of Italian and pop music make this Packer Avenue Italian one of Philadelphia's favorite stops before a game at the Vet or Spectrum. Though the ratings are not standouts, it may be the "best pre-game spot," with easy parking, party rooms, and nearly forty years of experience getting diners out in time for kick-, tip-, or face-off.

FOOD ROOM STAFF COST

Meiji-En

$32

Columbus Blvd. at Callowhill St., Philadelphia (215) 592-7100 on the Delaware Riverfront

This popular Japanese/American occupies a pier on the Delaware River, which accounts for its high ranking for view, and is extremely popular for its "outstanding Sunday brunch" with a buffet and an "excellent live jazz." The restaurant is so big it has a little of everything under its roof: a traditional dining room, a teppan-yaki room where you watch the chefs work, tempura and sushi bars, and a small garden with a waterfall. The down side: Some say the Japanese cooking is "marginal" and "too American."

Melrose Diner

$13

1501 Snyder Ave., Philadelphia (215) 467-6644
15th & Passyunk in So. Phila.

Got a hankering for gravy fries and creamed chipped beef on toast? No, you're not going mad, you just need to make a trip to the Melrose, the #1 favorite diner on the survey. Imagine a world where 30-plus year waitresses call you "hon," bring you meatloaf sandwiches, and apple pie in vanilla sauce, in what our voters call "a Philly landmark." It may be cop food, but you need to put your arteries to the test every once in a while.

Mel's Italian

$34

201 Jefferson St., Belmont Hills (610) 668-1712 on the Main Line

Our voters took the gloves off and let Mel have it in this year's poll. The biggest complaint was that it is "not worth the price," especially with the Manayunk restaurants just across the bridge. Other complaints: the decor is "tacky," the staff "acts like they're doing you a favor," and the food is "poorly prepped." "Overpriced for raw shrimp and bad wine," they advise Mel to just "give up."

Melting Pot

$25

8229 Germantown Ave., Chestnut Hill Hotel, Philadelphia (215) 242-3003 (at Southampton in Chestnut Hill/Mt. Airy)

The name of this Chestnut Hill reminds us that, while "melting pot" describes our great nation, it also describes that cheesiest of '60s fads: fondue. There is something fun, especially for couples, in the occasional dipping of hardened bread into a blend of three carefully melted cheeses. Maybe it's the funny forks, or the Sterno, or even the, um, fragrant aroma of the cheeses themselves. If you can figure it out, call us immediately.

Mendenhall Inn

$34

Rt. 52, Kennett Pk., Mendenhall (610) 388-1181 in Chester County

This dressy Chester County American-Continental—a "beautiful place, great for a special occasion"—gets its best scores among middle-aged and older voters. Reviewers deem the Colonial atmosphere, with either a pianist or harpist playing every night, "lovely" and "romantic," and the staff receives excellent marks. Crab dishes and prime rib are among the specialties on the traditional menu.

 = Superior = Excellent = Very Good

Mexican Post

$17

104 Chestnut St., Phila. (215) 923-5233 at Front St. in the Historic Area

Perhaps owner Nilesh Desai named this little spot in the Historic Area after the Mexican mail system to lower your expectations before you even walk in the door. Whatever his reasoning, he gets a wide array of reactions to the food, room and staff, ranging all the way from fair to average. It's "decent, cheap, and all the chips and salsa you can eat." P.S. "Good Margaritas."

Michael's

$23

824 S. 8th St., Phila. (215) 922-3986 at Christian St. in So. Phila.

This South Philly Italian may be only a year old, but already has a core group of fans. The regional and Tuscan cooking is certainly authentic: They serve "great game in season," and somewhere, Michael's mother is slaving away on the gnocci. "Delightful" raves one voter, but due to the small size and good food, you must reserve. "The best Tira Misu I ever had," adds one sweet tooth, "and I've had them all!"

Michael's Deli

$13

Rt. 202, Valley Forge Shopping Ctr., K. of Prussia (610) 265-3265 in Montgomery County

It's the kind of deli with "Jewish pickles right on the tables," in a dish, of course. You'll find good sandwiches, in goodly portions, and homemade salads (chicken, tuna, etc.), in your basic dump in the Valley Forge Shopping Center. With a huge beer selection, one doubly-negative voter comments that "no beer cannot be found there."

Michel's at the Latham Hotel

$35

17th & Walnut Sts., Philadelphia (215) 563-9444 in Center City

The imaginative cuisine is the draw at this mid-sized Center City California-French Bistro in the Latham Hotel on Rittenhouse Square. Voters are less impressed with the "unpredictable" service and the contemporary room than the "smart," "innovative" food and "fantastic presentation," especially of "the best desserts anywhere." The prices aren't too high for such creative cuisine, and prix fixe meals at lunch and dinner are an even better deal.

Mick's

$17

2500 Moreland Rd., Willow Grove Mall, Willow Grove (215) 830-8770 (Moreland & 611 in Montgomery County)

A few say this Willow Grove American is "fun with the kids," with "nice atmosphere" and "the best-trained staff." But enough others say the food is "consistently bad" to pull the score down to the "fair" range.

Mick's at the Bellevue

$18

Broad & Walnut, The Bellevue, Phila. (215) 732-7997 in Center City

This casual restaurant in the basement of the Bellevue seves what the management calls "Continental food with a Southern flair." Our reviewers cut to the chase: "Do not skip dessert." Mick's has a children's menu, crayons for the kids to play with, and good pub grub.

FOOD ROOM STAFF COST

Middle East

$23

126 Chestnut St., Phila. (215) 922-1003 at 2nd St. in the Historic Area

This Society Hill nightspot has been dishing out Middle Eastern food for nearly 40 years, and while some find the room "dingy," others laud the "consistently good food," "authentic ambiance" and the "biggest falafel sandwich in town—plus belly dancers" on Friday and Saturday nights.

Miller's Smorgasbord

$19

2811 Lincoln Hwy. E. (Rt. 30), Ronks (717) 687-6621
Rt. 30 — 2 miles East of Rt. 896 in Lancaster County

Our voters call this buffet "one of the best in the state," especially for the shrimp and chicken, and advise you to "load up." Lancaster County locals rub shoulders with visitors from all over, sampling freshly made dishes, even breakfasts and other dishes cooked to order. Not exactly a romantic, first date kind of place, but you probably want to know your partner pretty well before going back for seconds on dessert anyway.

Mill Race Inn

$33

183 Buck Rd. (Rt. 532), Holland (215) 322-2010 in Bucks County

The food, primarily hearty grilled meats, is "good," and the staff "pleasant" at this Holland American restaurant. But our voters really go for the "very nice atmosphere." There's a fireplace in this old converted grist mill, and even a piano player on weekends, but for a really special time, "get a table by the river," where you enjoy wonderful views of Mill Creek Falls.

Minar Palace

$10

1605 Sansom St., Phila. (215) 564-9443 at 16th St. in Center City

This Center City Indian is no palace—it's hard to find lower room ratings—but the north Indian food is "a real find for low-budget freaks, especially if you're a curry addict."

Minella's Main Line Diner

$12

320 W. Lancaster Ave., Wayne (610) 687-1575 on the Main Line

While most of the numerical votes gave this place lousy marks across the board, those voters who were moved to write comments were enthusiastic. "Good breakfasts" give way to "great homemade Italian food" (just the basics, running the gamut from manicotti to spaghetti). Families like it, students love it, and they get pretty busy at times. "For a diner, you can't go wrong," just about says it all.

Mirna's Cafe

$24

417 Old York Rd., Jenkintown (215) 885-2046
at West Ave. in Montgomery County

This Jenkintown Eclectic dazzles voters with top-notch salads, pastas and fresh fish, at relatively low prices. The service is more in keeping with the Euro-flavored music and flower-bedecked granite tables than the tiny, "cramped" room and bring-your-own-wine set-up, so some think it's "impeccable," others say it's "snooty."

Momi

$13

526 S. 4th St., Philadelphia (215) 625-0370
4th & South Sts. in the South St. Area

This unassuming little homestyle American in South Philly takes the "simple foods" and "does them well." "The staff is the greatest" raves one voter, creating a "friendly" environment in the "kitschy decor." One voter questions "why eat at a restaurants where everything they serve you could make yourself?" Because, another less accomplished cook answers, it's "great if you like Tang."

Monte Carlo Living Room

$51

2nd & South Sts., Philadelphia (215) 925-2220
in the South St. Area

No throw of the dice, this South Street (in location only) Northern and Southern Italian is a winner on all counts. Diners enjoy seeing the different cuts of meat and fish before ordering, and "always have a good meal, with great wines," thanks to Chef Nunzio Patruno. The over-40's nightclub upstairs adds that Monte Carlo feel. One of Philly's favorites, particularly where older patrons are concerned.

Montserrat

$20

623 South St., Philadelphia (215) 627-4224
bet. 6th & 7th in the South St. Area

While this little South Street restaurant has a French name, the food is American Eclectic. Many naysayers bring the averages down, but this place also has plenty of fans, from the Sunday brunch crowd to the little ones, who dig the coloring books. Voters "love the outdoor deck," and recommend this "groovy and hip" spot for lunch "by the weirdness of South Street." "Try Marcia's cheesecake."

Moonstruck

$28

7955 Oxford Ave., Philadelphia (215) 725-6000
at Rhawn St. in Northeast Phila.

The "good" food at this Provincial Italian in the Northeast has a flavor and richness that "can get you high," or so claims one extremely sensitive voter. The atmosphere, while decorated in a "whimsical" manner, is also "very romantic," so much so that more than one reviewer recommends against coming here with a large party. The staff, while good, is "too attentive" for some.

More Than Just Ice Cream

$11

1141 Pine St., Philadelphia (215) 574-0586
at 12th St. in Center City

This popular Center City dessert spot is famous for its "amazing," "memorable" Mile High Apple Pie (each contains 50 pounds of apples). Voters say the portions are "obscene—be sure to bring a friend," one reason it's popular for "post-date desserts—you can feed each other ice cream." The rest of the food gets mixed reviews.

FOOD ROOM STAFF COST

Moriarty's

$18

1116 Walnut St., Phila. (215) 627-7676 bet. 11th & 12th in Center City
This American Pub is popular before and after the theater because it has the "best burgers in town," "the greatest Buffalo wings," 16 beers on tap and service that will "get you to the theater on time." The main drawback: "The tiniest bathroom in the city."

Morton's of Chicago

$46

19th & Cherry Sts., One Logan Sq., Philadelphia (215) 557-0724 bet. Cherry & Ben Franklin Pkwy. in Center City
Number 8 overall for food in our book, and in the Top 20 of Philly's Favorites, it's the fact that Morton's is a top 10 business lunch and business dinner that tells the real story here. Though part of a nationwide chain, the "consistently good steaks" are called the "best in the city," even "the best steaks east of the Mississippi." And to go with them, "excellent drinks," including award-winning martinis. Cigar-friendly, one voter warns that it's "for expense accounters only."

Mother's

$27

34 N. Main St., New Hope (215) 862-9354
bet. Bridge & Randolph Sts. in Bucks County
This New Hope Eclectic changes with the seasons. Our voters tell us that the summer months bring on the tourists, and some of this restaurant's quality gets lost in the rush. We even hear that the weekend menu suffers from the same dilemma. When it's busy, it's "just alright," inspiring comments like "overrated." But when it's good, it's an "all-time favorite."

Mr. Martino's Trattoria

$24

1646 E. Passyunk Ave., Phila. (215) 755-0663
12th & Morris in So. Phila.
Here's the angle on this BYO South Philly Italian: You get simple, unadorned peasant food (polenta with sausage is the signature dish) in a building that once housed a hardware store. The dining room and menu both are small but well crafted, and you won't get hammered by the prices. One voter sums it up: "Family run, good home-cooked Italian food, low prices."

Mrs. Marty's Deli

$12

Rt. 320, Lawrence Park Shopping Center, Broomall
(610) 359-1996 in Delaware County
323 E. Gay St., Sharpless Sq., W. Chester (610) 701-9575 in Chester Co.
Busy and big, this Broomall American deli, with Jewish-style (though non-Kosher) items is coming up on its 10th anniversary. Most of our voters call the food "average" or better, served in what are called "healthy portions." "The sandwiches are great"—no surprise—but lots of people think it should be cheaper, especially with the "indifferent" staff and the dumpy decor.

 = Superior = Excellent = Very Good

Murray's Deli

$14

285 Montgomery Ave., Bala Cynwyd (610) 664-6995
at Old Lancaster Rd. on the Main Line

It's the battle of the Jewish Delis, on Montgomery Avenue in Bala Cynwyd. On this side, Murray's, that's "always good, if a little pricey," vying for the "top deli in the area." On the other side, Hymie's. "Murray's has the better bagels," say voters, but it's down to personal taste. Who will win? On our survey, Murray's—but we'll let the "rude waitresses" fight it out.

Museum Cafe

$11

33rd & Spruce Sts., U. of Penn., Philadelphia (215) 898-4089
in University City/W. Phila.

A little anthropology, a little archaeology, and a little American food. What could be better? Well, the food for starters. The kitchen in this Museum restaurant seems to be in need of updating, and folks certainly don't dig the staff. However, it is an unique setting, one that will keep the extremely curious happy for a day trip.

Museum Restaurant at the Phila. Museum of Art

$20

25th St. & Ben Franklin Pkwy., Philadelphia (215) 763-8100
in the Art Museum Area

"Surprise," say our voters, for though the buffet at this American restaurant, located in the Philly Art Museum, is provided by a large, familiar catering corporation, it is actually pretty good. In addition to lunch, it has a "great buffet dinner on Wednesday nights." Although the place is "relaxed and pleasant" it still "hasn't found its identity."

Mustard Green

$21

622 S. 2nd St., Philadelphia (215) 627-0833
bet. South & Bainbridge Sts. in the South St. Area

Our voters think very highly of this Nouvelle Chinese in the South Street area, so much so that one Romac Reporters says it's "as good as Susannah Foo's, without the hype." Well, maybe that's carrying things a little too far, and for those who are used to always carrying out their Chinese meals, they might be surprised at the above-average-for-Chinese prices. Whatever their opinions, our voters agree, the food is always good since "everything is FRESH!"

My Thai

$19

22nd & South Sts., Phila. (215) 985-1878 in S.W. Center City

This bite-sized, casual Thai in Southwest Center City has earned a reputation for "good food in a lousy neighborhood." The unimpressive room is a drawback for older voters, but everyone agrees it's one of the city's best ethnic buys for the money, especially the fixed price dinners for under $15.

FOOD ROOM STAFF COST

Nais Cuisine

$30

13 W. Benedict Ave., Havertown (610) 789-5983, at Darby Rd. in Delaware County

So many Romac Reporters said this Main Line French/Vietnamese was "the best-kept secret around" the word must have leaked out. Others assure us that "despite being discovered, it's still a favorite." "You can't beat the duck," we're told, but all the offerings are "divine," "fresh and delicious," the "best food for the money anywhere." Voters are glad that, after a decade, "it's still BYO."

Napoleon Cafe

$29

2650-52 E. Somerset St., Philadelphia (215) 739-6979 bet. Richmond & Thompson in Port Richmond

This place is large enough not to have a Napoleon complex, though it still has a split personality: Downstairs is a bustling coffeehouse, serving "excellent pastry" to the younger side of the crowd, while upstairs, a more elegant restaurant takes greater pains to please, serving very good Contemporary American cuisine. Stick your hand in your shirt and "make the drive to Port Richmond—it's worth it."

Narberth Natural Foods

$10

231 Haverford Ave., Narberth (610) 667-7634 on the Main Line

Don't be scared off by the name, or by the fact that this spot is in the back of a health food store. This tiny shop blends flavors from Mexico, Italy and the Middle East to produce very inexpensive, good and unusually flavorful healthy meals. You'll find "fantastic" tuna salad, with minced carrots and tahini, stuffed into a pita.

Nella Cucina

VOTE

Easton Rd. & Keswick Ave., Glenside (215) 887-9020 in Mont. Co.

This little cafe, located a couple of doors down from the Keswick Theater, opened at the end of our survey period. A few Romac Reporters have sampled it, and they say this "friendly neighborhood spot" with "interesting pasta and pizza" looks promising. There's also a patio for when the weather's nice.

New Corned Beef Academy

$12

1605 Walnut St., Phila. (215) 561-6222 at 16th St. in Center City

Hand-carved turkey and "the best corned beef in the city limits by far" make some people say this Center City deli is "as good as if not better" than the original Corned Beef Academy. Several note, however, that it's "expensive for just a sandwich."

New Deck Tavern

$13

3408 Sansom St., Philadelphia (215) 386-4600 bet. Chestnut & Walnut in University City/W. Phila.

Named after a new deck, this Irish Tavern could use a new approach to the American food they serve. But, as long as you pick dishes that go with cold beer and TV sports, you should do fine at this "smoky dive," that caters mostly to "jocks and students."

New Delhi Indian

$16

4004 Chestnut St., Philadelphia (215) 386-1941
at 40th St. in University City/W. Phila.

The numbers agree with the voters: This is "the best of University City's several good Indian restaurants." "No glamour awaits you in this storefront, but pamper your taste buds with a trip," says one voter, and you can also pamper your wallet with the inexpensive "incredible buffet" at lunch and dinner.

Nifty Fifties

$12

1356 E. Passyunk Ave., Philadelphia (215) 468-1950
10th & Reed Sts. in So. Phila.
2491 Grant Ave., Philadelphia (215) 676-1950 in Northeast Phila.
1900 MacDade Blvd., Folsom (610) 583-1950 in Delaware County

Voters visit these loud, bright burger shacks (the original is in South Philly) for "nostalgia, great burgers," the "excellent milkshake selection" and "a nice change of pace" (reviewers are divided over the merits of the pork barbecue). It's among the top-rated places to take kids, in large part because "you could feed a small army on $20."

94th Aero Squadron

$29

2750 Red Lion Rd., on the runway of the Northeast Phila. Airport, Philadelphia (215) 671-9400 (in Northeast Phila.)

The location, overlooking the runway of the Northeast Airport, and the World War I French farmhouse atmosphere are the selling points for this Northeast Philly Continental. Unfortunately, voters say the food is so-so and patrons "get rushed through the meal." Still, it's a "fun place to take out-of-state friends."

Noah's

$24

225 Washington St., Conshohocken (610) 941-9200 at Fayette St. in Montgomery County

Here's something different—a riverfront restaurant that's not on the Delaware. This Conshohocken American Eclectic, floating on two barges in the Schuykill, is decked out with carousel animals in a Noah's Ark theme, creating a "quaint, fun novelty" that's "different—I would go back." Remember that you're getting "bargain food among the factories" and you won't be disappointed.

Noodle Heaven

$18

220 S. Broad St., Phila. (215) 735-6191 at Locust St. in Center City

Voters find "top-notch dim sum" and "great peanut noodles" at this Center City Chinese next to the Bellevue Hotel; some stumbled on it and discovered a "great pre-theater place" (remember to BYO). The drawbacks: plain decor and an open kitchen with poor ventilation, making the smell of the cooking sometimes "overpowering."

FOOD ROOM STAFF COST

North Star Bar

$20

2639 W. Poplar St., Philadelphia (215) 235-7826
at 27th St. in the Art Museum Area

"Not your standard bar fare" say voters of this Art Museum Area Contemporary American, which might be best known for "great local rock bands" but is equally popular for its casual Asian and Tex-Mex menu. Infrequent visitors say it "seems like a local hangout and definitely a dive, but fun." Regulars say "whenever we go away, North Star is the place we love to come back to."

Ocean Garden

$20

9423 Race St., Philadelphia (215) 928-0451
10th & Race Sts. in Chinatown

Though they have neither a garden nor an ocean on premises, the fresh fish and lobster tank still makes a good centerpiece to this Chinatown Cantonese and Szechuan, specializing in seafood dishes. Try the Friday night lobster special.

Ocean Grille

$25

7700 City Ave., City Line Shopping Ctr., Phila. (215) 473-1400
in the City Line Area

This City Line Area American (with an Italian flair) Seafood grill has "very good" food, even if we do hear complaints that the portions are a bit "skimpy." Casual and calm, they have six wines by the glass, the ingredients are always fresh, but beyond the "great" menu, not much stands out about this place, unless you notice the "slightly tacky" nautical decor.

Ocean Harbor

$21

1023 Race St., Philadelphia (215) 574-1398
bet. 10th & 11th in Chinatown

"The food, the crowd, the noise," make dining at this Chinatown Chinese "as close as you can get to Hong Kong without leaving Philadelphia." The "great dim sum" at Sunday brunch is the highlight for most voters, who also seem to appreciate the improving decor.

Odette's

$37

S. River Rd., New Hope (215) 862-2432 at Rt. 232 in Bucks County

This New Hope Continental is popular with baby boomers, who like the historic building's fireplace, antiques and view of the Delaware River. The food receives good scores, but some say the "nice menu" is "kind of bland."

O'Hara's Fish House

$23

3900 Chestnut St., Philadelphia (215) 349-9000
at 39th St. in University City/W. Phila.

A new owner and chef are trying to improve the grades for this nautical-themed University City Seafood spot, adding all-you-can-eat crab and shrimp specials. Crab cakes remain a popular choice.

Old Brauhaus

7980 Oxford Ave., Philadelphia (215) 728-9440 in NE Phila.
Creeping up on its thirty year anniversary, this Northeast Philly German American has remained a relative outsider to the city's restaurant scene. The food is "very good," "the best German food in the area" (it is also one of the only Germans around). This authentic spot disproves the general rule that the food can't be good if the restaurant has "beer" in its name.

Old City Coffee

$8

221 Church St., Philadelphia (215) 629-9292
bet. 2nd & 3rd, Market & Arch Sts. in the Historic Area
With the "best coffee shop atmosphere," this cozy, European-style cafe is only open for breakfast, brunch and tea time. "Don't let Starbuck's tell you different—THIS is coffee," say fans of this "reliable spot." Good for a cheap caffeine pick-me-up, this joint makes our Top 10 lists for best coffeehouse and best espresso/cappuccino.

Old Guard House Inn

$34

953 Youngsford Rd., Gladwyne (215) 649-9708
1 blk. off Rt. 23 on the Main Line
The "very Main Line" Old Guard has enjoyed this Gladwyne seasonal American and Continental for the last 140 years, though the structure first went up more than 200 years ago. While there is some disagreement over the food, "this place wins for historic dining—it is not just a facade!" "Too costly for a neighborhood place," writes one voter, and he's right: this is something special. One swinging reviewer comments that this place was "built in the 1700s, and the clientele is the same age." Shame on you, young man.

Old Mill Inn

$28

York & Horsham Rds., Hatboro (215) 672-6593
in Montgomery County
This 18th-century grist mill in Hatboro has been turning out meals for half a century now, but some swear they've "never had a bad meal." Its Continental menu and early bird specials prompt cries of "a senior citizen's delight," but as is often the case, it actually ranks higher with younger voters, and the food isn't all that stodgy—grouper in a horseradish crust with dill sauce is a popular dish. With a kids' menu and rooms ranging from a romantic nook with low ceilings and exposed beams to an enclosed porch with a view of the Pennypack Creek, it's clear why the Old Mill Inn keeps rolling along.

Old Original Bookbinder's

$41

125 Walnut St., Philadelphia (215) 925-7027
at 2nd St. in the Historic Area
The Old Original owners stopped binding books in 1865 and opened this big, Historic Area seafood and steakhouse, often called a "tourist trap," though the owners say they're trying to turn the place around. The gripe heard most often is that it is "extremely overpriced for average food," and though unaffiliated, voters recommend you "try the 15th Street Bookbinders for food, and the Chestnut Hill location for atmosphere." Still, some say it's a must for visitors.

FOOD ROOM STAFF COST

Oregon Diner

$15

302 Oregon Ave., Philadelphia (215) 462-5566
bet. 2nd & 3rd in So. Phila.

This South Philly diner's food isn't first-rate, even by diner standards, but the selection is varied—Italian, Greek, classic diner fare, even Chinese—and the portions are satisfying. "Slop, but good slop," say the voters. With table jukeboxes, "great rice pudding" and, some say, "lots of smoke," the atmosphere is authentic. But the service isn't—not one reporter complains about mean waitresses.

Ortleib's Jazz House

$21

847 N. 3rd St., Philadelphia (215) 922-1035
3rd & Poplar Sts. in Northern Liberties

The spicy Cajun food at this Regional American and Eclectic restaurant takes a back seat to the "great live jazz," served up to an appreciative crowd. Folks recommend it for a "sophisticated first date," again for the music and not necessarily for the "beer and good sweet potato fries." Don't get us wrong—the food is good, and this place makes for "a great all-around evening out."

Otto's Brauhaus

$23

233 Easton Rd., Horsham (215) 675-1864
at Pine Ave. in Montgomery County

"Brauhaus" means "Brew House," and this cozy traditional German place in Horsham has many features usually found in larger brauhauses: fresh imported beers on tap plus a wide variety in the bottle, and a good buffet of traditional dishes that get high marks for cuisine from der fatherland. And, the waitresses wear "dirndls," or, literally translated, "St. Pauli Girl outfits."

Outback Steakhouse

$24

610 Old York Rd., Jenkintown (215) 886-5120 (Montgomery Cty.)
3420 Tillman Dr., Bensalem (215) 633-8228 in Bucks County
561 Glen Eagle Sq., Glen Mills (610) 558-0644
in Delaware County
1162 Baltimore Pk., Olde Sproul Shopping Ctr., Springfield
(610) 544-9889 in Delaware County

This Steak chain is clearly popular—why else would so many voters complain so bitterly about long waits (up to two hours at times) for a table? Many feel the steaks are "good for a chain" and rave about the whole, batter-dipped "bloomin' onion." Others say it is just "Rustler with an accent" and "way overrated." The restaurant's dinner-only hours make it "not very user-friendly." The concensus? "Good steak fun" after a "cows to slaughter" wait.

Overtures

$32

609-611 E. Passyunk Ave., Phila. (215) 627-3455
5th & South Sts. in So. Phila.

Light sauces and a very up-to-date menu characterize this "marvelous" South Philly European (primarily French) restaurant. Called "a favorite little hideaway," this "memorable" little spot is made even more romantic (and inexpensive) with a bring-your-own wine or beer policy. Whisper this "best kept secret" in your neighbor's ear.

 = Superior = Excellent = Very Good

Oyster Bar at the Marshalton Inn

$24

Rt. 162, West Chester (610) 692-5702 at Sugarsbridge Rd. in Chester Co.

The rustic renovated barn gives a false clue about what's inside—this West Chester American-Seafood spot is a fun place for "great food and entertainment"—with different bands most nights. The food is "always good" though the menu is "somewhat static."

Pace One

$36

Thornton & Glen Mills Rds., Thornton (610) 459-3702 in Chester Co.

Once again, our voters tell us that the setting is the real draw at this historic Thornton spot. The American fare has a few standouts, including "great snapper soup," but there is a "sameness" to the menu that some diners find "tiresome." The 250-year-old restored barn, with a fireplace, soft music and private rooms, is what keeps our voters coming back.

Paganini

$25

72 W. State St., Doylestown (215) 348-5922 at Rt. 611 in Bucks Co.

A planned move across the street may pump up the room and ambiance rating, but as far as the food and staff, this Doylestown Italian earns "very good" marks. Though the choices on the menu may be "limited," the ingredients are always "fresh" and "high quality." What is professional service to some, becomes "snobbish," and "trying to impress" to others.

Painted Parrot Cafe

$11

209-211 Chestnut St., Phila. (215) 922-5971
at 2nd St. in the Historic Area

This Society Hill coffee shop is one of the survey's top dessert spots, a "cute place" that's "a must after Ritz movies." Wednesdays feature an all-you-can-eat dessert buffet; the themes change weekly, but voters recommend you "try chocoholic night," the third Wednesday of each month.

Palace of Asia

$25

285 Commerce Dr., Fort Washington (215) 646-2133
1/2 mile off Rt. 309/PA Tpk. in Montgomery County

You have to go to Montgomery County for one of the top rated Indian restaurants in the area: just look at those scores! And, with "amazing ambiance," the "authentic food" draws many "natives of India" to this place. In addition to these votes of authenticity, they have a great bargain lunch buffet, and Indian Kosher dishes available. It's "worth the drive."

Palladium

$26

3601 Locust Walk, Philadelphia (215) 387-3463 (DINE)
at 36th St. in University City/W. Phila.

You get "incredible ambiance, especially in the summer," at this University City International. In the summer, they have "unparalleled outdoor dining," with a "great view" of the university campus. In the winter, it becomes a cozy spot, with a "lovely fireplace and collegial atmosphere," though some call it "dark." Students find it "a bit pricey" —but you're paying for more than just the food.

FOOD ROOM STAFF COST

Palm

$41

200 S. Broad St., The Bellevue, Philadelphia
(215) 546-PALM (546-7256) at Walnut St. in Center City

Romac Reporters say this archtypical steakhouse is Center City's "best place to see and be seen," which might explain why it ranks as the survey's best spot for both business meals and eavesdropping. Steak, naturally, is the star; everything, including vegetables, is a la carte. Though the ambiance is relaxed, the high-powered crowd strikes some as "pretentious," and several complain of "uncomfortable chairs."

Pamplona

$23

225 S. 12th St., Philadelphia (215) 627-9059
at Locust St. in Center City

This Center City tapas bar gets very good marks for its Spanish food, and many rhapsodize about the authentic decor: It has "fantastic art work." Younger voters find the atmosphere exciting; older ones are more likely to call it noisy. Be aware that eating tapas is the ultimate in grazing—the "perky" staff will bring one appetizer-sized portion as soon as the last is done, so some people say the service is slow, while others complain of being rushed.

Panorama

$35

14 N. Front St., Penns View Inn, Philadelphia (215) 922-7800
at Market St. in the Historic Area

The "incredible wine selection," housed in the largest cruvinet machine in the world, is the draw at this Historic Area Northern Italian. Wine spectators are pleasantly surprised by the "satisfying and pleasing" food, and professional service in a room that gets a bit loud at times. With many different wine tasting programs, one voter claims it's "like being in Firenze," though you pay in dollars, not lire.

Paolini's

$20

758 W. Haverford Ave., Bryn Mawr (610) 525-9994
at Bryn Mawr Ave. on the Main Line

After almost 40 years, this Main Line Italian still serves mostly old-fashioned favorites at old-fashioned Italian food prices.Though the grades are just fair, some voters have found "simple but great pasta" and "good food at a low price." The best night to visit is Saturday, when grandmother makes homemade lasagna.

Passage to India

$22

1320 Walnut St., Philadelphia (215) 732-7300
at Juniper St. in Center City

The Center City location, "Indian food at its best" and room ratings (and prices) higher than most Indian spots lead to comments like "the best Indian in the city, but you'll pay for it." A few dissenters sniff that the food is "very mild." The BYO policy keeps the tab within reason, and live music is featured—piano on weekends, sitar on Wednesdays.

 = Superior = Excellent = Very Good

Passerelle $39

175 King of Prussia Rd., Radnor Racquet Club, Radnor (610) 293-9411 bet. Lancaster Ave. & Radnor-Chester Rds. on the Main Line

This dressy Radnor Continental-American's "wonderful food" and "beautiful presentation," along with its strikingly landscaped setting in a "nice romantic spot," make it "one of the best on the Main Line"—"expensive and worth it." Unlike many top-flight places, it scores just as high for its "attractive, excellent and tasteful service." P.S. A few say the large, open room "lacks privacy."

Pasta Blitz by Lamberti $20

212 Walnut St., Phila (215) 238-0499 (2nd & Walnut in the Hist. Area)

Convenient to the Ritz 5, this Italian restaurant specializing in lighter fare certainly gets blitzed by consumer traffic, though diners disagree over the consistency of the food. Those familiar with the other Lamberti locations find the food wanting, but what it lacks in creativity is made up for in large portions and a comfortable atmosphere.

Pat's King of Steaks $8

1237 E. Passyunk Ave., Philadelphia (215) 468-1546 9th & Wharton Sts. in So. Phila.

"Make sure you have your order ready," say fearful clients of this Cheesesteak capitol of the world. "You've gotta love a place where you're afraid to order," says another. But tough cooks aside (or maybe it's the long-term health risks our voters fear), this No. 2 (yes, number TWO) favorite cheesesteak joint, with no indoor seating, "made cheesesteak famous." "There's always a line, even at 3 a.m. in the rain," we hear, and "they're always there when you need them." It's a piece of Philadelphia that stays in your arteries for a lifetime.

Pattaya (fka Sweet Basil) $21

4006 Chestnut St., Philadelphia (215) 387-8533 at 40th St. in University City/W. Phila.

Bargain-hunters flock to this University City Thai not just for its innovative cuisine—"light and different," "kind of Ameri-Thai" with French influences thrown in—but for its inexpensive prix fixe lunches ($7.95) and dinners ($9.95). The mood is casual, reservations are essential.

Pepper Mill $13

Rt. 352 & Paoli Pk., East Goshen (610) 692-0100 in Chester Co.

This Chester County hoagie and pizza spot earned top-10 Romac honors for its cheesesteaks. "Heaven is a chicken cheesesteak with a chocolate shake."

Peppers Cafe $14

2528 Haverford Ave., Ardmore (610) 896-0476 on the Main Line

"Everything is in cream sauce" at this former Main Line burger shack, now a mostly-takeout northern Italian, where patrons can sit at a tiny counter and watch the chef concoct dishes like penne with crabmeat and porcini. "Great takeout, good food, not low fat."

= Good **= Fair** **[no rating] = Poor**

FOOD ROOM STAFF COST

Persian Grill

$20

637 Germantown Pk., Lafayette Hill (610) 825-2705
at Butler Pk. in Montgomery County
"Authentic Iranian food" is only one attraction at this Lafayette Hill Middle Eastern. The "extraordinary flower garden in the front," replete with waterfall and pond, draws just as many compliments. The inexpensive lamb, beef and seafood entrees might just broaden your international taste buds.

Philadelphia Fish & Co.

$24

207 Chestnut St., Philadelphia (215) 625-8605
bet. 2nd & 3rd. in the Historic Area
Some folks go for the "innovative approach to fish dishes" at this seafood and New American restaurant, that is often called "the best," at least in Olde City. The neighborhood feel (read "plain") has some patrons expecting larger portions or lower prices, but most voters look to the food, the "good wines by the glass," and a generally "friendly waitstaff," especially the bartenders, and leave this place well satisfied.

Phillips Mill, Inn at

$42

2590 N. River Rd., New Hope (215) 862-9919 in Bucks County
This little New Hope Inn is one of the best Country French spots in the book. You get "the feel of Southern France," with "great food and great ambiance." Those who have spent the night at the charming inn, in addition to partaking of the very good breakfast, call it the "most romantic in the Philadelphia area," and recommend you "sit outside in the summer." BYO.

Philly Rock Bar & Grill

$14

1400 S. Delaware Ave., Phila (215) 463-5771 (Reed St. in S. Phila.)
Twelve TVs with sports playing nonstop. Ten cent wings on Monday night. "48 beers on tap." Tuesday Happy Hour. Kids eat free Monday to Thursday, 4-8 p.m. "It is cheap." Ice cream. Hey, even the rest of us, who like to speak in complete sentences will enjoy it.

Phil's Tavern

$18

931 W. Butler Pk., Blue Bell (215) 643-5664 (Montgomery Cty.)
"This place may be nothing to look at, but man-sized meals await," writes one hungry Jack of this Italian American pub in Blue Bell. This family place has enjoyed more than 50 years of serving good food to hungry patrons, in a setting that has been around for four times that long. Everything is simple and good, and "flavorful, too. Far above standard pub grub."

Pikkle's Plus

$10

113 S. 16th St., Phila. (215) 561-0990 (16th & Sansom. in Ctr. City)
An old-fashioned, breakfast-and lunch-only Jewish Deli in Center City, that you'd think would have gained more fans in its fifteen years of business. The best they get is "a good lunch spot," but most voters think it's a "dive." There's hope, however—the owner is putting in new booths, new tables and a new floor.

= Superior = Excellent = Very Good

Pink Rose Pastry Shop $10

630 S. 4th St., Philadelphia (215) 592-0565
at Bainbridge St. in the South St. Area

Here is the pastry and dessert spot that places highest in our overall food ranking, and no wonder. Our voters "wish all their 'extra' calories would come from here." You may have to wait, and confections of this quality don't come cheap, but for "perfect" cappuccino, "pastries done with pleasure," and "even low cholesterol for passover," it's "always the perfect dessert."

Pipersville Inn $31

Rts. 413 & 611, Pipersville (215) 766-7100
in Bucks County

The Pipersville Inn is in Pipersville, of course, and so are its "very good" Country-style American dishes. The open, friendly setting keeps a steady stream of fans visiting this out of the way spot, "an all-around good value for a Saturday evening." Reservations are recommended on weekends, and with these prices, you don't pay the piper.

Pleasant Peasant $27

1500 Locust St., Philadelphia (215) 893-9100
15th & Locust in Center City

The name of this Center City American Eclectic is catchy but not accurate—"more than pleasant and certainly not peasant," one reporter croons. Many like the "interesting selections" on the "unusual menu"—"you can't go wrong . . . from appetizers to dessert" (don't skip the "superior" chocolate souffle cake). Some note the "gorgeous presentation," others observe that "portions can be small," making the food "not really worth the price." The consensus: "A little artsy-fartsy but a good meal."

Plumsteadville Inn $39

Rt. 611 & Stump Rd., Plumsteadville (215) 766-7500
in Bucks Co.

The combination of early American decor and Continental cuisine makes this historic spot in Central Bucks a winner. The six dining rooms, two with fireplaces, earn excellent grades; the food, which features seafood with local vegetables and specialty sauces on a menu that changes daily, isn't far behind. Voters recommend "for a warm, cozy atmosphere," "go when they have a piano player."

Pollo Rosso $22

8229 Germantown Ave., Philadelphia (215) 248-9338
at Southampton Ave. in Chestnut Hill/Mt. Airy

This Chestnut Hill Italian, where "pasta and pizza rule," scores highest among families with kids. Voters love the "eclectic pizza," grilled and rotisserie-cooked entrees, good microbrew selection and "the best bread pudding," all at "very reasonable" prices. All that's enough to make most people overlook the noise, occasionally slow service and long waits.

FOOD ROOM STAFF COST

Portofino

$22

1227 Walnut St., Phila. (215) 923-8208 (bet. 12th & 13th in Ctr. City)
Voters give the food and decor at this Center City Italian-Continental just so-so ratings, but the reasonable prices and friendly service make this a popular spot for before-theater dinners. Reservations essential.

Positano

$30

801 Sproul Rd., Springfield (610) 543-6644 at Springfield Rd. in Delco.
21 W. Lancaster Ave., Ardmore (610) 896-8298 across from the Ardmore movie theater on the Main Line
The Delco member of this Italian pair is "a fun BYO place," and while the room won't bowl you over, the staff gets good marks. Some find the menu too traditional, but regulars say the kitchen is "very accommodating about food preparation." The younger Ardmore Positano has a liquor license while offering the same kind of seafood-oriented Italian menu as its sibling.

Primavera

$26

2nd & South Sts., Phila. (215) 925-7832 in the South St. Area
Reviewers say this casual sister to the Monte Carlo Living Room serves "wonderful food," particularly "great pasta" and "the best linguine pescatore." The exposed-brick, trattoria-style room a "lovely place," that is so small you should "be prepared to meet the diners next to you."

Primavera

$25

384 W. Lancaster Ave., across from Wayne Farmer's Market, Wayne (610) 254-0200 (at Conestoga Rd. on the Main Line)
Reactions to this Wayne Northern Italian are definitely mixed, with a few fans giving the place top marks, but just as many saying they "did not have a good experience." The prices are "reasonable."

Primavera Pizza Kitchen

$22

7 E. Lancaster Ave., Ardmore (610) 642-8000 at Station Ave. on the Main Line
The converted bank setting is the star at this Italian Pizza spot in Ardmore. The "really great ambiance" includes a "fun and lively" crowd and "fantastic" trompe l'oeil designs in a "pretty" room that some think is "the best decorated eating spot anywhere." The menu doesn't live up to the decor, and gets uneven results from voters. But prices are low—and "what a place to eat pizza!

Priori's

$16

1000 Wolf St., Philadelphia (215) 339-9358 at 10th St. in So. Phila.
This South Philly spot focuses mainly on provincial and Northern Italian dishes, much to the liking of the few people who can get into this tiny place. The "old family atmosphere" is just that—62 years old and counting. "Great mussels" are part of the "very good" menu. This place could use a sprucing up, more room, and more cheerier staff. But it is just that atmosphere that makes this feel like a find. Reservations essential.

 = Superior = Excellent = Very Good

Pronto

544 York Rd., Center Point Place, Warminster (215) 672-3300
at Street Rd. in Bucks County
"Pronto" may be the first word Italians yell into the telephone, but, according to our reviewers, it's not the last word in Italian food at this large restaurant in Bucks County. When you take into account some of the amenities, from the cheap prix fixe dinners, to the interesting historic memorabilia on display, when you're on the road this may be just what's called for.

Que Pasta!

4460 Main St., Philadelphia (215) 482-4892
Green Ln. in Manayunk/Roxborough
This Manayunk Italian deli impresses voters with its jumbo ravioli, garlic and basil pasta and tomato paradiso sauce. "Delicious food at a great price" earns high marks, but the poor score for ambiance reflects a room that "needs a face lift."

Quickie Chickie

9th & Federal Sts., Phila. (215) 467-1234 in So. Phila.
This South Philly spot offers a local alternative to the ubiquitous bird joints for rotisserie chicken and freshly prepared vegetable dishes. Voters praise the "very good cornbread" and "quality birds." Do the 3 a.m. cheesesteakers spurn nearby Pat's and Geno's in order to reduce their cholesterol intake? Not yet.

Quissett

$28

379 Lancaster Ave., Haverford (610) 896-0400
at Haverford Sta. Rd. on the Main Line
Scores were all over the voting scale for this Haverford Mediterranean. While it may cost less than comparable Center City places, with an early bird prix fixe menu, what is an overall "delightful" restaurant to some voters, who think "the new chef does a good job," as many others say it "used to be better before the latest change." We also hear griping about inconsistency and small portions. As an upscale Mediterranean, Quissett might miss it.

Rachael's Nosherie

$10

120 S. 19th St., Phila. (215) 568-9565 19th & Sansom in Center City
This little Jewish/American Cafe has a few fans, who mainly appreciate the accessibility and "good value" of the limited menu, but the majority of our voters don't think this place deserves high marks. Could be the fact that they don't have any china, or that they're closed on Sundays, but we think it has something to do with the fact that "homemade" isn't always to everyone's taste.

FOOD ROOM STAFF COST

Ralph's Italian

$22

760 S. 9th St., Phila. (215) 627-6011
bet. Catherine & FitzwaterSts. in So. Phila.
The family that has run this South Philly standby for nearly a century knows how to keep voters happy—big portions of traditional fare (mussels, greens and eggplant parmesan all are recommended) in a bustling, everyone-is-family atmosphere. This kind of food strikes some as "average at best," but far more consider Ralph's "an orgasmic culinary experience."

Randazzo Pizza

$12

1826 South St., Philadelphia (215) 546-1566
bet. 18th & 19th in the South St. Area
Voters say this South Street pizzeria is inconsistent, but others "recommend the veggie special—it's loaded with goodies."

Rangoon Burmese

$16

145 N. 9th St., Phila. (215) 829-8939 bet. Cherry & Race in Chinatown
Looks like "the Jewel of Chinatown" is about to steal away. But not to worry, this "delicious cross between Indian and Thai, with friendly family management" is merely moving across the street, and is hoping to keep the same phone number. No matter where you find Rangoon, it's worth it: after all, Columbus discovered America looking for its spices.

Ray's Coffee Shop

$18

141 N. 9th St., Philadelphia (215) 922-5122
bet. Cherry & Race Sts. in Chinatown
Expecting chrome, and a tattooed counterman named Ray? Guess again. "Thirtysomething meets Chinatown" at this Taiwanese and Chinese spot, that is the number two coffeehouse on our poll. While the food is "good and cheap," it takes a back seat to the individually prepared siphon coffee, well regarded as "the best $5 cup of coffee in town."

Reading Terminal Market

$11

12th & Arch Sts., Philadelphia (215) 922-2317
in Center City/Chinatown
While the Reading Terminal Market is not any one restaurant, many diners consider it a single destination, so we thought we'd let our voters write about it as a collective. And, just like we try to do with our guidebook, our voters only reported on what they like—and according to them, there's plenty to like. The consensus is that it's "the best Philadelphia place to take guests to shop and for lunch," with scores of vendors of every food type, from greengrocers to sandwiches, to Soul Food and Mexican—and great desserts—"you name it, and the Terminal probably has it." It is "one of Philadelphia's treasures," though "confusion reigns supreme!"

= Superior = Excellent = Very Good

Regatta Bar & Grille at the Phila. Marriott West $24

Rt. 23 & Fayette St., W. Conshohocken (610) 941-5600
in Montgomery County

You probably guessed that this Hotel American has a nautical theme working. Voters consistently report that the food is only average, with room and staff not much better. However, we suggest a second look, since they recently enclosed the glass deck, making happy hour "uplifting" to some. Breakfast and brunch are serviceable, but we suggest the Regatta for a drink after work.

Rembrandt's $26

741 N. 23rd St., Philadelphia (215) 763-2228
at Aspen St. in the Art Museum Area

After canvassing a large group of voters, we found that, though this place doesn't pull down the ratings of an old master, it does keep them coming back for more American and Continental food. Still, many voters say it's "the best in the Art Museum Area," for a "romantic cocktail," "great bar," good brunch and lovely view of the Philly skyline.

Rendezvous $23

503 W. Lancaster Ave., Spread Eagle Village, Wayne
(610) 971-0851/0852 on the Main Line

"Super food for a great price." Our voters say that this International spot may well be "the best BYO on the Main Line." Mediterannean and Middle-Eastern dishes dominate the menu, and one voter simply moans "that rack of lamb." They try to give the place a romantic feel, but it's really casual and informal. How romantic can you get in a mini-mall called the "Spread Eagle Village?" Don't answer that.

Restaurant & Bar $22

18-22 W. Gay St., West Chester (610) 431-0770
at High St. in Chester County

Unfortunately, the fish, pasta and cajun dishes at this bar and restaurant in Chester County are not quite as creative as its name, but many of our voters were perfectly satisfied. It's a "fun," "great hangout for young couples," who don't seem to mind the sometimes "slow service."

Restaurant School $25

4207 Walnut St., Philadelphia (215) 222-4200
at 42nd St. in University City/W. Phila.

Dining at this University City culinary arts school can be a Jekyll-and-Hyde experience—it's a laboratory for would-be chefs still learning their craft, so "you never know what you'll get." Some report the French cuisine is "a pleasant surprise," others call it mediocre. The "elegant" room overlooking a "beautiful atrium" gets very good grades, but scores for service are as uneven as those for food. With such reasonable prices, though, adventurous Romac Reporters consider the trip "risky, but worth it."

FOOD ROOM STAFF COST

Rhapsody's

VOTE

25 S. Broad St., Lansdale (215) 362-5669
at Rt. 63 in Montgomery County

Our voters wax poetic about this two-year-old Continental in Lansdale. The "Nouvelle cuisine is flavorful and creative," they say. The staff receives "excellent" marks for professional and attentive service. And the room, though small (it seats 55), also gets high marks for its restored 1800s setting. Unfortunately, when the local's on time, the "adjacent railroad tracks can detract from the dining experience."

Rib Crib

$18

6333 Germantown Ave., Philadelphia (215) 438-6793
Washington & Johnson in Chestnut Hill/Mt. Airy

Romac Reporters rank this Mt. Airy Barbecue spot the survey's best, and say its pit-barbecued chicken and ribs with "positively addictive hot sauce" make it the No. 1 Sleeper. If it's such a hideaway, by the way, what are all those celebrities' pictures doing on the wall?

Rib-It

$20

52 S. 2nd St., Philadelphia (215) 923-5511
2nd & Chestnut in the Historic Area and many other locations

Proof that you can't quantify taste: while most agree that this chain is "dark," like a "dive," and the high number of voters consistently gave the ribs and other bar food "fair" marks, it has still managed to become number one for ribs on our poll. Football fans and gourmands of all sizes appreciate the "best all-you-can-eat baby back rib specials" on Monday nights—"go ahead, be a pig!" Neophytes appreciate the "scrumptious" sampler of this place's "excellent ribs."

Rib Rack

$21

425 Township Line Rd., Elkins Park (215) 379-0300
in Montgomery County
6900 Bustleton Ave., Philadelphia (215) 338-9399 (in NE Phila.)

"Great food, simple style, great salads" is the credo of these popular and inexpensive barbecue joints. Their "great Buffalo wings and baby back ribs" are referred to as the "best," maybe even "in the USA," with "sauce that is out of this world." Whatever the criteria, they're good enough to make the Top 5 for ribs in the front of the book. P.S. While the Northeast location has a liquor license, the Elkins Park Rib Rack is a BYO.

Ritz-Carlton Lobby Lounge

$29

17th & Chestnut Sts. at Liberty Place, Philadelphia
(215) 563-1600 in Center City

The tables in the very public lobby of the Ritz-Carlton offer, ironically, a great deal of privacy—one reviewer says it's "my favorite place to gossip, unhurried and elegant—you can linger for hours." Perhaps the best time to do it is afternoon tea, "elegant in a WASPy sort of way" as you nibble on "great pieces of tiny food." You can just drop in—they don't take reservations—making it a great stop for "a Christmas treat" during the shopping season.

 = Superior = Excellent = Very Good

River Deck Cafe & Dance Club

$24

4100 Main St., Phila. (215) 483-4100 (Shurs Ln., Manayunk/Roxborough)

So the food's not that great. It doesn't keep a large crowd of all ages (under-30s make up most of them) from eating big portions of "only fair" Continental cuisine and bar food. They need it, to keep their strength up for the "great dancing afterwards." Ladies beware: "the ladies' room is in a difficult location—up a winding staircase."

Rizzo's Italian

$15

21 E. Glenside Ave., Glenside (215) 887-2909
at Easton Rd. in Montgomery County

This Glenside pizzeria and family-style Italian turns 50 this year, and while the decor hasn't changed, ownership did in the '80s, and some old fans say it's "just a shadow of its former self." It remains "Glenside's gathering place" and a "great stop before a show at the Keswick," partly for its "good neighborhood pizza" (No. 4 in the survey), and also because "the staff is great"—"friendliest service anywhere."

Rocco's Famous Italian Hoagies

$8

200 S. Broad St., Food Court at the Bellevue, Philadelphia (215) 772-1220 at Walnut St. in Center City
Reading Terminal Market, Phila. (215) 238-1223 in Center City

These hoagie shops get uncommonly high marks for sandwiches that start with "great rolls" and are built with fresh, gourmet-quality ingredients. Reviewers suggest the "chicken a la Rocco hoagie," and anything with roasted peppers.

Rock Lobster

$26

221 N. Delaware Ave., Philadelphia (215) 627-ROCK (627-7625)
at Vine St. on the Delaware Riverfront

Our voters took several cracks at this Lobster, located on the Delaware riverfront, with a "great view" of the Delaware and the Ben Franklin Bridge. Romac reviewers found the food "plastic," though the pickup scene and the entertainment were both Top 10 winners. Bring a roving eye, and try the good rock lobster salad. Closed in the winter.

Roller's

$27

8705 Germantown Ave., Phila. (215) 242-1771
at Bethlehem Pk. in Chestnut Hill

Romac Reporters flock to this Chestnut Hill Modern American for fresh, healthy, "unusual cuisine" that's "always worth the wait." They like the open kitchen, but note that the small room gets "too warm in hot weather" and say "elbow room is at a premium."

Ron's Ribs

$17

1627 South St., Phila. (215) 545-9160 (bet.16th & 17th So. St. Area)

Chef/owner Ron Washington first had to learn the secret of how to prepare the ribs at this South Street Barbecue/Soul Food spot before he could buy it. For the last ten years, he has come through with perhaps "tastiest ribs on the east coast," #3 on Romac's barbeque list. You can bring your own beer or wine, but most prefer takeout.

FOOD ROOM STAFF COST

Roosevelt's Pub & Pizzeria

$14

2222-16 Walnut St., Phila. (215) 636-9722 (bet. 22 & 23rd in Ctr. City)

The food is just fair in this Center City spot, located in what used to be the Roosevelt Hotel. The draws are the pool tables and "an arcade the size of a football field."

Rosario's

$24

13 S. Morton Ave., Morton (610) 544-2744 at Rt. 420 in Delaware Co.

This Delaware County family spot's "menu is always new and exciting," mixing Italian and Modern American influences. Locals say it's "a favorite for married couples' date night," perhaps because it's fairly inexpensive and, if the baby sitter cancels, the restaurant is well-equipped to handle kids.

Rose Brier Inn

$25

8828 Frankford Ave., Philadelphia (215) 333-8800
Academy Rd. exit off I-95 in Northeast Phila.

While the American food at this big restaurant in the Northeast may not be knocking them dead, they have added Murder Mystery nights to their roster of activity-based dining. Other common events are weddings, rehearsal dinners, showers and graduation parties. "Friendly" and "fast service" actually has voters just coming here for dinner.

Rosebud's Cafe

$19

8201 Germantown Ave., Philadelphia (215) 248-0990
at Hartwell Ln. in Chestnut Hill/Mt. Airy

Outdoor dining that ranks among the city's best is the claim to fame for this Chestnut Hill Eclectic. Some like the "great noshie food" and "good desserts," but others say the "heavy-drinking crowd is not that interested in the food."

Rose Tattoo Cafe

$28

19th & Callowhill Sts., Phila. (215) 569-8939 (in the Art Museum Area)

With five dining areas, this very popular Art Museum area Modern American offers atmosphere to suit any mood. Voters call it "the ultimate pseudo-New Orleans getaway" and love the "relaxing jungle" ambiance of the plant-filled second floor. The kitchen's internationally influenced "haute country cuisine" and "amazing presentation" score very well, and it's among the top 10 for desserts. But it's clearly the "upbeat, refreshing" "fun and sophisticated" atmosphere that makes voters call it "a great date place" and among the top 10 for conversation.

Rose Tree Inn

$37

1243 Providence Rd., Media (610) 891-1205
Rts. 1 & 252 in Delaware County

You get "fireside dining with entrees prepared by an Austrian Chef" at this highly-rated restaurant in Media. Chef/owner Robert Rottensteiner prepares Continental specialties, including crab dishes and the "best double lamb chops," to an appreciative crowd, served by an "attentive," "very good" staff. Reserve in advance, wear a jacket and tie, and get a seat by one of this inn's five fireplaces.

Royal Scot

$27

400 Bridge St., Phoenixville (610) 983-3070 at Rt. 23 in Chester Co.
If you're in the mood for haggis, you'll have to look elsewhere. This Phoenixville highlander specializes in American and British pub food, from burgers and fries to Shepherd's and steak & kidney pies. More than 100 years old, the rooms "transport you to London," and are split up into a main dining room, a pub, and a large private room. Keep it simple, for "while the food may not be fit for royalty," the bar, with its large selection of imported beers and drafts, "is a blast."

Ruby Tuesday

$17

1250 Baltimore Pk., Springfield Mall, Springfield (610) 543-7509
Rt. 320 & Baltimore Ave. in Delaware County
Franklin Mills Mall, Phila. (215) 281-2791 in Northeast Phila.
Granite Run Mall, Media (610) 891-6711 in Delaware County
Some say this corporate-owned American is "Bennigan's—the way it should be." That would mean a "great salad bar," of course, with specially flavored dressings like the raspberry vinaigrette, "good Bloody Marys" and fun little touches like honey butter for your rolls. But the Bennigan's benchmark cuts both ways, and the sandwiches can be "sort of greasy." What is "reasonably priced" to some is "a bit pricey, for a mall" to others.

Russell's 96 West

VOTE

96 W. State St., Doylestown (215) 345-8746
at Main St. in Bucks County
This upscale, elegant Doylestown Contemporary American (with a very Continental attitude) distinguishes itself among the far-suburb, historic setting establishments. The atmosphere is "intimate," and "very romantic," pulling down top marks as does the "excellent" service, that is professional but not fussy. And the food—"a work of art," say some, with the proper "attention to details and flavors." The 6-course degustation menu is a treat for the self-indulgent, and you must remember to call ahead.

Ruth's Chris Steakhouse

$44

260 S. Broad St., Phila. (215) 790-1515 at Spruce St. in Center City
With a Top 100 food score, and a Top 20 rating in Philly's favorites, especially for business dinners, this nationwide steakhouse chain is so good, some of our reviewers think "they should establish a dress code" (to keep out the riff-raff). With many individual dishes mentioned as "the best" (since everything on the menu is a la carte), many consider the steaks to be "the best in the city." With these kinds of crowds, however, we get the inevitable complaints about overbooking, long waits at the bar, and high prices. Whatever Ruth's Chris charges, it hasn't kept the crowds away.

Saigon

$18

935 Washington Ave., Phila. (215) 925-9656 (at 10th in S. Phila.)
This South Philly Vietnamese has been "consistently great over the years," its food "very authentic," "convenient and cheap." The room provides humble but "comfortable surroundings," and the "nice people" who run the place provide "great service."

FOOD ROOM STAFF COST

Saladalley

$13

1001 Baltimore Pk., Springfield Sq., Springfield (610) 328-5880 bet. Rts. 320 & 420 in Delaware County
Suburban Square, Ardmore (610) 642-0602 on the Main Line

The ratings don't look spectacular, but the high vote count for this American shows that plenty of people still stop by, especially in Springfield, where the salad bar has grown into a hot and cold buffet. "For $5.99 on weekdays, it's the best buy in town," voters say, though they don't much care for the service or the "cafeteria atmosphere."

Saloon

$49

750 S. 7th St., Philadelphia (215) 627-1811
bet. Fitzwater & Catherine Sts. in So. Phila.

This South Philly Italian is "still one of the best in town," "a great spot for locals and tourists" that garners some of the highest food and service scores in the survey, as well as a spot among the top 10 favorites. It wins raves for its "fine service," antique-filled decor and "fresh ingredients, fine cheeses and wines." "Fantastic chops" and "enormous steaks" stand out on a "large menu, well-cooked with many daily specials." "Great dining if you can handle the expense."

Sampan Inn

$15

8 Brookline Blvd., Havertown (610) 446-2188 at Darby Rd. in Delco

One voter asked that we "don't tell anyone" about this multi-regional Chinese, that most agree is "the best Chinese restaurant in the Suburbs," but we have big mouths. We'll need those mouths when we visit this place in Havertown, where "enormous servings" are the norm, and with such low prices and lowfat options on the menu, we can eat to our heart's content. One diner warns, "the lines are out the door, and the food is out of this world."

Sam's Grill

$13

2 Jenkintown Commons , Jenkintown (215) 572-8805
Old York & Wyncote Rds. in Montgomery County

People visit this Jenkintown grill when they want "great hamburgers," chicken and ribs that are "a cut above fast food." The "great little place" is "always packed," and customers stay entertained by the "crazy people who work there."

Samuel Adams Brew House

$18

1516 Sansom St., 2nd fl., Philadelphia (215) 563-2326
bet. 15th & 16th Sts. in Center City

The Sam Adams label can now read "Brewer, Patriot, Restaurateur." The food, "marginal" to some, "surprisingly creative" to others, is not the center of attention here. It's the microbrews that offer a satisfying distraction for the basic "bar crowd."

Samuels

$37

503 W. Lancaster Ave., Wayne (610) 687-2840
at Eagle Rd. on the Main Line

Once again, the "elegant French country dining room" and "very good" service have outscored the food at this Main Line American. Half our reviewers describe a "delicious and interesting menu," while the other half are less impressed, prompting some to call Samuels "overpriced." P.S. Try the $19 "spectacular" champagne Sunday brunch.

San Carlo

$35

214 South St., Phila. (215) 592-9777 bet. 2nd & 3rd in the South St. Area

Our voters argue over whether the food at this Southern/Central Italian is "very good," or "excellent." What they do agree on is the authenticity of the cuisine, calling it "real food from Italy," courtesy of the Trusone family. With a "casual" atmosphere, consisting of paintings and mirrors on the walls, and a "staff with personality," this is another little gem on South Street.

Sang Kee Peking Duck House

$16

238 N. 9th St., Phila. (215) 925-7532 bet. Race & Vine in Chinatown

"I still love this hole-in-the-wall," writes one reviewer. "If they could only do something about the grease on the floor." Ahh well, "dirty but cheap," that doesn't exclude this family-owned spot from the title of "the best and most innovative Chinese restaurant in Chinatown." And our reviewers mean it; just look at those ratings.

San Marco

$36

27 City Ave., Bala Cynwyd (610) 664-7844
bet. Bryn Mawr & Bala Aves. in the City Line Area

While many voters give this Classic Italian in Bala Cynwyd top marks, dissenters pull the averages down to "good." But here is a suburban restaurant from the old days: you dress up, leave the car with the valet, and sit in a quiet and dark room by the fireplace, to be served by "snooty waiters." While this "old reliable has gotten better with time," it has also gotten more expensive, and to some it is "overpriced."

Sansom Street Oyster House

$22

1516 Sansom St., Philadelphia (215) 567-7683
bet. 15th & 16th Sts. in Center City

This Center City Seafood house is in its twentieth year of serving "very fresh seafood" to appreciative business lunch diners and to a dinner crowd that skews to the older set. Whatever the crowd, the price tag is low for the location and the reliable quality of the food. While there are few innovations, the fish at this "always dependable" spot is "absolutely fresh." "Go for lunch," writes one mathematician. "It's half the price of dinner."

FOOD ROOM STAFF COST

Scampi

$26

2312 Garrett Rd., Drexel Hill (610) 284-3333
at Lansdowne Ave. in Delaware County
Prices are reasonable at this Drexel Hill Italian, which specializes in seafood. The family-oriented staff is well-equipped to deal with kids—one reason it scores highest among thirthysomethings.

Scoogi's Classic Italian

$22

738 Bethlehem Pk., Flourtown (215) 233-1063
in Montgomery County
Business lunch? In Flourtown? So say our voters of this fresh Classic Italian restaurant, calling the food "good," the staff "very pleasant," and "quick." That shouldn't deter families from enjoying Scoogi's, for it serves moderately priced dinners, including kids' specials. Family owned, it is comfortable and popular.

S.C. Toland's

$20

500 W. Ridge Pk., Conshohocken (610) 828-2727
at Butler Pk. in Montgomery County
Area diners, interested in simple, Italian/American and seafood dishes, point their cars down Ridge Pike toward this family-style, kid-friendly restaurant in Conshohocken. With a "rustic" atmosphere, good crab cakes, it's "always good and reasonable," especially to our easier-to-please reviewers.

Seafood Unlimited

$18

270 S. 20th St., Phila. (215) 732-3663 (bet. Spruce & Locust in Ctr. City)
The price is right at this unpretentious, fresh fish market in Center City. The kind of place with "blackboard specials, and no frills, " it's "FUN, with an elbow-to-elbow crowd." Some say that "out-of-town guests enjoy the informality," but as far as we can tell, so does everybody else. Watch the tanks: Maybe you'll see your next meal.

September's Place

$24

642 Baltimore Pk., Springfield (610) 544-1230 in Delaware Co.
Though best-known for catering, the Delaware County American/Continental also drew attention for its "great champagne Sunday brunch," inexpensive lunch buffet and early bird specials and what some voters call "surprisingly delicious food." But scores are all over the map; detractors say the fare is "banquet-esque."

Serrano/Tin Angel

$22

20 S. 2nd St., Philadelphia (215) 928-0770
bet. Market & Chestnut in the Historic Area
While this place purports to serve "International home cooking," our reviewers advise you to "stick with the Continental fare," since some of the other, far Eastern dishes "lack their spicy character." But while the food may not burn your insides, this cozy Olde City spot, with its brick walls and wood burning stove, will warm your outsides. Upstairs at the Tin Angel, you'll find "great inexpensive entertainment," with "terrific live music."

 = Superior = Excellent = Very Good

Seven Stars Inn

$38

Rt 23 & Hoffecker Rd., Phoenixville (610) 495-5205 in Chester Co.
As far as we know, four stars is as high a rating as a restaurant can get, so we consider this name wishful thinking. Wishes do come truc, according to our voters, at this large, formal Phoenixville restaurant. Don't be alarmed by the price tag, a bit high for an out-of-towner; you get "very generous portions" of "unbelievable prime rib and lobster tails" and other American favorites, that celebrate a time when cholesterol was a word that only dieticians and hypochondriacs used. Call and ask about their special wine tastings and cigar dinners.

1700 Lombard Cafe

$19

17th & Lombard Sts., Philadelphia (215) 772-1700 in Center City
The young professional crowd has quickly taken to this Center City newcomer, where you can bring your own wine to go with the "good comfort food with an elegant twist." "A great neighborhood addition," voters say, with "good food in a cute spot" decorated in a bicycling motif. The low prices make it a "great value."

Seville (fka Galileo's)

VOTE

17th & Spruce Sts., Phila. (215) 735-4611 in Center City
This is one tough place for our voters to get a read on. It opened after our survey last year as Galileo's, with an Italian menu. It is now Seville, with a Spanish Tapas menu. "What's all the fuss for?" If you find out, let us know.

Sfuzzi

$25

1650 Market St., Liberty Place, Philadelphia (215) 851-8888 bet. 16th & 17th Sts. in Center City
Business lunchers appreciate the breezy atmosphere and dependable food, while socializers frequent this place for an after work drink, placing Sfuzzi in the Top 10 in both categories. The rest of our voters, on the other hand, see it as a "pickup place for yuppies, though the food is good." While some say it is "dependable," particularly for "good brunch," just as many think Sfuzzi is "overrated."

Ship Inn

$28

Rt. 30 and Ship Rd., Exton (610) 363-7200 on the Main Line
"Old in atmosphere, with small rooms and fireplaces," this Regional American in Exton is celebrating 200 years of serving Philadelphia pubgoers in style. While the kitchen never gets any raves, it has a core of diehard fans, and many others coming around to the cause: "It gets better every visit."

Shiroi Hana

$23

222 S. 15th St., Phila. (215) 735-4444 (bet. Walnut & Locust in Ctr. City)
The sushi is just great at this Center City Japanese with traditional decor. Freshness is the key to great sushi, but they also have a handle on the other disciplines of Japanese cooking in this well-ordered environment. "Crowded on weekends," you probably want to call ahead. One well-meaning sociopath writes it's also "great for eavesdropping."

FOOD ROOM STAFF COST

Shogun

$23

1009 Arch St., Phila. (215) 592-8288 at 10th St. in Chinatown
You don't have to show your gun, or your credit card either, at this Chinatown Chinese and Japanese restaurant. With all the usual ethnic specials and low prices, there are few standouts here: they have a "laid back separate bar area," and an unusual "teapot soup." All in all, it's best known for being "undiscovered."

Siam Cuisine

$22

925 Arch St., Philadelphia (215) 922-7135
bet. 9th & 10th Sts. in Chinatown
4950 York Rd., Buckingham Green Shopping Ctr., Buckingham (215) 794-7209 (in Bucks Co.)
2124 S. Eagle Rd., Village at Newtown (215) 579-9395 in Bucks Co.
Many reviewers agree that the "first Thai restaurant in Chinatown" is still the best. They have a loyal group of fans that have tried the rest, and say this is the "best Thai food in Philly," "hotter than any Thai around (sometimes TOO hot!)." The other locations throughout the area, though somewhat "Americanized," are "still good," with house specialties like the Thai spiced coffee.

Siamese Princess

$22

36 E. Lancaster Ave., Ardmore (610) 896-2755
at Rittenhouse Pl. on the Main Line
A recent move to Ardmore throws the room rating out the window, but the Thai food at this little Main Liner still earns consistently above-average marks. "The move from Manayunk is still worth the hunt," says one voter, for what another calls "the best dumplings in town." Though we hear the new decor, French with pretty wallpaper and table linens, is an improvement, one diner thinks "it's not quite the same yet."

Sign of the Sorrel Horse

$52

4424 Old Easton Rd., Doylestown (215) 230-9999
in Bucks County
The French/Continental cuisine may be good at this Bucks County restaurant, though the history seems more interesting than the food: Built during the Revolutionary War, it housed the offices of General Lafayette, and the mill supplied flour for Washington's troops. Now the kitchen may not supply enough food to the tables: "I left hungry!" complains one diner of the portions.

Silk City

$14

435 Spring Garden St., Philadelphia (215) 592-8838
at 5th St. in Northern Liberties
If we had included a fifth voting category—sentimental value—this place would have pulled down a top score. That helps explain why the food ratings are spread so evenly from good to bad, as are the room and staff votes. It's a stainless steel diner that looks like something out of a movie set, with a '50s-style American menu that may not bear up to today's healthy standards. So what? Kick off your shoes and try to dance off some of those fat calories in the adjacent lounge.

Silk of Siam $20

614 W. Lancaster Ave., Bryn Mawr (610) 527-0590
at Penn St. on the Main Line

"Best Asian BYO on the Main Line—friendly service, good Thai food" sums up the reviews of this small Bryn Mawr restaurant: our more poetic voters say there is "a delicate mingling of spices." BYO usually means rock-bottom prices, so some Romac Reporters think this Silk's "a bit pricey."

Silk Road $20

414 Lancaster Ave., Devon (610) 964-7625
on the Main Line

If you want a fatty hit of MSG, go somewhere else. A few rave that this Main Line Chinese serves "excellent, low fat creations," with good service, and, even more unusual for a Chinese place, "good coffee and dessert." The iffy ratings are probably due to the fact that all this is not what people expect from a Main Line Chinese, but if you want to save your arteries, drive your car to the Silk Road, and BYO.

Singapore Kosher Vegetarian $16

1029 Race St., Philadelphia (215) 922-3288
bet. 10th & 11th in Chinatown

Placing a solid 6th on our Top 10 list for Vegetarians, this Chinatown Multiethnic draws on flavors from throughout Southeast Asia, much to the delight and satisfaction of our voters. "The meals are tasty, the portions huge, and the staff"—very good, by all accounts—"is attentive." Folks recommend the "sesame bananas," and other "unusual vegetarian dishes."

Sitar India $14

60 S. 38th St., Philadelphia (215) 662-0818
bet. Chestnut & Market Sts. in University City/W. Phila.

While the food does not aspire to greatness, this is a nice, inexpensive little alternative when you're in the University City area. Like many Indian spots, the all-you-can-eat, prix fixe lunch and dinner buffets are the real bargains, making it tough to spend more than ten bucks a person. Kids and infants are welcome, though the food might be too spicy for their little palates.

16th St. Bar & Grill $21

264 S. 16th St., Philadelphia (215) 735-3316
bet. Spruce & Locust Sts. in Center City

"Welcome back, 16th. St; good riddance, Mango Bay," say Romac Reporters about this Mediterranean spot's brief sail into the Caribbean. While most voters are "glad to see they went back to the old menu," that some call "consistently inventive and fun," food ratings are all over the charts, "sometimes good, sometimes disappointing." Still, the averages are solid for a neighborhood bar, leading us to believe the new owner/longtime manager Michael Stemmer has shaken out the wrinkles.

FOOD ROOM STAFF COST

Skippack Roadhouse

$37

4022 Skippack Pk., Skippack (610) 584-4231
at Mench Rd. in Montgomery County

Some folks love this Montgomery County American Continental, but a restaurant with this much hype and a food rating that falls well below the room and staff tallies, is bound to be "disappointing" to many. Still, the historic setting is pretty to look at, the weekend jazz combo is pretty to listen to, and the view is pretty, from the room that overlooks a babbling brook.

Smokin Sam's Italian Grill

$18

417 Germantown Pk., Lafayette Hill (610) 941-4652
at Joshua Rd. in Montgomery County

Don't worry about secondary smoke, Sam is too busy smoking the ribs, ham, turkey and chicken for a big crowd at this Lafayette Hill "locals hangout." The menu seems to have a split personality, that keeps everyone happy, for in addition to the heavy side, including "great ribs" and beer, Sam's also serves lighter, Cal-Ital fare.

Society Hill Hotel

$16

301 Chestnut St., Phila. (215) 925-1919 at 3rd St. in the Historic Area

The location, in the heart of Independence Historical Park, guarantees this bed-and-breakfast hotel bar a steady audience for its "basic" menu of Philly-style favorites. The jazz piano attracts a nighttime crowd, and voters say it's a good stop "before or after your movie at the Ritz." One problem: a "rude" staff that prompted one reporter to wonder, "If they don't care, should I?"

Solo Mio

$21

232 Arch St., Philadelphia (215) 625-9820
bet. 2nd & 3rd Sts. in the Historic Area

While this "nice, unpretentious Italian" restaurant doesn't win any prizes for its "good Italian food," diners who have only sampled the appetizers, pastas and main courses owe Solo Mio a second look, especially where desserts are concerned: what one voter calls "amazing cheesecake," another says is "amazing, amazing, amazing cheesecake (and turtles)." But, as the Sinatra and Mathis on the stereo continue to age, some think it's "not as good as it used to be."

Sonoma

$28

4411 Main St., Philadelphia (215) 483-9400
at Gay St. in Manayunk/Roxborough

The most impressive number we got on this Manayunk California-Italian isn't in the ratings: it's the huge number of people who have visited the place and have offered their comments, widely varied though they are. What is an "in" place to some is "fake LA attitude" to others, and what is "excellent and fun, seven days a week" turns into a "smoky pickup scene, at least later in the evenings." Whatever your take, the now-famous vodka bar has helped define the scene in Manayunk. N.B. reserve the "single table on the back patio, all by itself, quiet and wonderful."

= Superior = Excellent = Very Good

South Philly Bar & Grille $21

2026 S. 12th St., Phila. (215) 336-8833 at Mercy St. in So. Phila.
With a friendly, local atmosphere, this neighborhood South Philly Italian "joint," specializing in seafood, keeps 'em coming back for the big portions, welcoming staff ("better for regulars," like anywhere else), may have the "best food for the value." One reviewer says it's "like eating in Aunt V's clean kitchen," though we wonder if she'd ever decorate with so much "red & velvet."

South Street Souvlaki $16

509 South St., Philadelphia (215) 925-3026
bet. 5th & 6th Sts. in the South St. Area
It would be a challenge to find Greek food that's this authentic and good in a room that was any less plain. It's "very cheap," according to voters, with standout dishes like the marinated octopus appetizer, rotisserie chicken, and of course the souvlaki. "For the amount of money spent, this is a great place."

Spaghetti Warehouse $16

1026 Spring Garden St., Philadelphia (215) 787-0784
bet. 10th & 11th in Northern Liberties
"Warehouse is the word," voters warn of this mega-sized Italian in Northern Liberties. The "humble" food is "mass-produced," but the collection of old artifacts is impressive, particularly the trolley car that's been refitted for dining. Those who gripe that the kitchen's output "tastes like summer camp food" should remember that kids love summer camp; because the Warehouse is "cheap and fun," it's among the Top 10 spots for children. One voter recommends that you "take the kids and eat later."

Spiga D'Oro $30

831 Providence Rd., Primos (610) 284-2225
in Delaware County
The Providence Square Shopping Center location isn't the best, which might be why so may people chose this Delco Italian as their top sleeper. Penne with vodka and marinated eggplant earned special mention; you can bring your own wine or beer, which keeps the prices reasonable, moving one voter to call it "our favorite BYO."

Spirit of Philadelphia $36

Lombard Cir. at Columbus Blvd., Philadelphia (215) 923-1419
on the Delaware Riverfront
What is a "moving experience" to some (literally—this is a cruise ship that takes you around Philadelphia's harbor) is more like an evening-long "Love Boat" wannabe to others. Spirit is known more for the entertainment and lovely views than for the "heavy" Continental menu. While some think it's a bit of a "waste," others say the "live show is worth every penny." Reserve, and show up on time.

FOOD ROOM STAFF COST

Spotted Hog

$28

Rt. 202 & Street Rd., Lahaska (215) 794-4030
in Bucks County

This Peddlar's Village Contemporary American aims at a young crowd with an impressive list of microbrewery beers, and live rock music (Thursday through Saturday nights). Earlier in the day, it's a good stop for breakfast or lunch with the kids "to fortify you for all that shopping."

Spring Mill Cafe

$37

164 Barren Hill Rd., Conshohocken (610) 828-2550
River & Barren Hill Rds. in Montgomery County

With a slight North African and Vietnamese influence to the primarily French Provençal menu, this former country store in Conshohocken is some diners' "favorite place on Earth." While the atmosphere may be "cramped," it is "very French, with indoor and outdoor dining." It's a bit pricey for a BYO, and there are recent complaints that "it used to be better—has gotten old and dusty instead of rustic and rural."

Spring Mill Country Club, Inn at

VOTE

80 Jacksonville Rd., Ivyland (215) 675-6000
in Bucks County

While the lounge and golf course are for members only, the Italian American restaurant is open to the public, and thank heavens for that. Voters deem the food "very good," and the country club atmosphere "excellent" (it was renovated last year). The staff befits a restaurant where a jacket and tie are required after 6pm: formal, neat and professional. Call ahead, and bring small bills for the valet.

Stazi Milano

$24

West & Greenwood Aves., Jenkintown Train Station, Jenkintown (215) 885-9000 in Montgomery County

Once again, room and ambiance win out at this refurbished Jenkintown Train Station, done to the hilt in high Art Deco style. All that limestone creates "a candidate for soundproofing," which can "distract from dining" but is nevertheless to younger voters a "fun atmosphere," and most agree the food is "consistently good." Whoever said "real trains coming and going" outside "feels like Italy" has never waited at the real Stazi Milano.

Steak & Ale

$25

2224 Roosevelt Blvd., Trevose (215) 638-9442
in Bucks County

Overall, our voters recommend you visit this national chain outpost in Trevose, but while they suggest you go early, they don't necessarily think you should go often. "Great early bird specials" are one enticement; a "decent salad bar" and "fine steaks" add up to a good value. Once regular dinner time hits, "be prepared to wait, even with reservations." Says one discouraged diner: "It's better than it sounds."

 = Superior = Excellent = Very Good

Stephen's

$33

105 Shurs Ln., Philadelphia (215) 487-3136
at Cresson St. in Manayunk/Roxborough

Chef Kenneth Ulsh came from Totaro's, and many of the customers followed him to this Manayunk mecca of "very good" Italian and Mediterannean food. In contrast, the atmosphere is that of an English bar/restaurant: you enter at the bar level, and go upstairs to the dining rooms, built by the owner himself. Some say it's "quaint," but at least that means "comfortable," and overall it's "outstanding—especially the waiters, who know their stuff."

Stoxy's Steaks

$10

Pine Valley Ctr., Philadelphia (215) 677-5208
at Philmont Ave. in Northeast Phila.

This steak shop ensures a large, loyal clientele by cutting its own steaks and serving only what's fresh every day. Add "clean atmosphere" and you have a sandwich spot fans say "beats Pat's and Geno's every day of the week."

Striped Bass

$53

15th & Walnut Sts., Philadelphia (215) 732-4444 (in Center City)

"A class act," "this year's 'in' place" wins our Top Business Dinner category, and peppers many other Top 10 lists. The room is "georgeous:" Most Romac Reporters gave the decor a perfect rating. The kitchen earned a top 25 score, and Striped Bass is also one of Philly's favorites. The most typical of the reams of comments calls it "the most beautiful and overpriced restaurant in town." "Creative dishes" and "beautiful presentation," not to mention the professional staff, have backed up Striped Bass's big P.R. machine, but with this much hype, a few are bound to be somewhat "disappointed."

Strolli's

$14

24 W. Baltimore Ave., Lansdowne (610) 259-5962
at Lansdowne Ave. in Delaware County

That's right, this is the same restaurant that was on Dickenson Street in South Philly for almost seventy years, until last September. Now it has moved its family style to Lansdowne. No matter where they go, the Italian food remains "very good," but sentimental voters miss Mr. Strolli's birthday serenades.

Sugar Mom's

$14

225 Church St., Philadelphia (215) 925-8219
in the Historic Area

This Historic Area American occupies a building that was once a sugar refinery. It now features an "incredible beer selection," including a few custom-brewed for the tavern, in a room full of games and amusement park artifacts that give it "a lot of character." The food gets just fair grades, but voters approve of the "very reasonable prices."

FOOD ROOM STAFF COST

Sun Valley Pizza Co.

$12

838 Montgomery Ave., Narberth (610) 667-0500 at Iowa Ave. on the Main Line
In the top 10 for pizza in our guide, this Narberth joint may well have the secret to "fast food for the nineties:" with two kinds of nonfat cheeses, lean meats, "great sauce and crust," and "cool toppings," the food is satisfying and heart-healthy. They even have "good hoagies." Remember that a "good" rating can translate to "great low-cal food."

Susanna Foo

$40

1512 Walnut St., Phila. (215) 545-2666 (bet. 15th & 16th in Ctr. City)
Throw out your preconcieved notions about Chinese food before entering this "elegant," "innovative," even "magnificent" haute Chinese on Walnut. More than half the voters gave Susanna their top rating for "mouth watering Asian cuisine," with staff and room ratings that outstrip most other Philly dining spots. Still, some hold on to old ideas, and by comparison, they say it's "expensive," with relatively "small portions." According to Susanna Foo's fans, it blows other top restaurants away—"quietly the best in town."

Swann Lounge at the Four Seasons

$33

1 Logan Sq., Philadelphia (215) 963-1500 in Center City
Voters heartily recommend the Light Continental menu as a lower-priced alternative to the Fountain, "the best dining value with luxurious surroundings in town." The Sunday buffet brunch is a standout, but one of the best deals in the city is the weekend evening special—a $15 Viennese dessert buffet and dance music played by a jazz combo.

Sweet Potato Cafe & Bakery

$11

4 W. State St., Media (610) 891-1460 at Jackson St. in Delaware Co.
This Media Eclectic is best known for its muffins, cakes and pies, "incredibly rich and always delicious." Its soups, "great takeout salads and breads" attract a lunch crowd that includes a lot of vegetarians.

Tacconelli's Pizza

$15

2604 E. Somerset St., Philadelphia (215) 425-4983 bet. Richmond & Aramingo Sts. in Port Richmond
One voter exclaims that this Port Richmond spot has "the best pizza in the world! Guaranteed!" Everyone seems to agree: Tacconelli's is the #1 pizza on our poll, and places a remarkable 26th for food overall. "Horrendous" waits are due to the fact that pizzas are prepared one at a time. But with these ratings, and specialties like "garlic and spinach white pizza," the wait is well worth it. On weekends especially, you must call ahead to reserve your dough.

Taco House

$9

1218 Pine St., Phila. (215) 735-1880 bet. 12th & 13th in Center City
Frequented almost exclusively by young voters, who say it's "hip, cheap food," "good when you are hungry and you don't have lots of money." More discriminating palates say, "Don't bother. Everything is swimming in a nondescript brown sauce."

 = Superior = Excellent = Very Good

Tai Lake $21

134 N. 10th St., Phila. (215) 922-0698 bet. Race & Cherry in Chinatown
"Talk about fresh," Romac Reporters rave about this Chinatown Chinese. Aquariums in the lobby are filled with live fish, lobsters, dungeness crabs, even eels and frogs—your dinner is still swimming when you walk in. "Most of the Chinese restaurant owners eat here," one voter confides. Another advises: "Nothing beats the barbecued scallops." Open until 3:00 a.m. daily.

Tandoor India $15

106 S. 40th St., Philadelphia (215) 222-7122
in University City/W. Phila.
If it's not "West Philly's best Indian," at least it's the most heavily trafficked, with lots of voters telling us about the "nice buffet" and great "all-you-can-eat" specials here. That's nothing new, especially for a neighborhood Indian. The food is generally regarded as better than most. Though "not extremely private," it's kid-friendly, and plenty cheap.

Tang's $25

429 South St., Philadelphia (215) 928-0188
bet. 4th & 5th Sts. in the South St. Area
A core group of fans give owner Ranee Tang mixed reviews for his South Street Chinese restaurant. With a good selection of wines by the glass, classical and jazz music in the background and reservations a must, some voters say it's "second only to Susannah Foo for Chinese." Others disagree, citing "amateurish service," and food that is trying to be "too gourmet." If you find what the fans enjoy, like "nectarine chicken and dumplings, 10+, best in Philadelphia," Tang's "can be superb!"

Tang-Yean $16

220 N. 10th St., Philadelphia (215) 925-3993
bet. Race & Vine in Chinatown
While the menu of healthy Chinese options has stayed the same, "new owners" cast a pall over the ratings and comments of this old Chinatown favorite. We say give Tang-Yean a chance; in some voters' opinion, it has "the best Chinese food in the city," that won't make you fat.

Tapas $24

1176 N. 3rd St., Philadelphia (215) 922-2376
at Girard Ave. in N. Phila.
"We need Spanish restaurants," moans one global gourmand, "but the location of this place is so bad!" That aside, this Classic Spanish has managed to please diners with "gourmet Spanish dishes, with lingering memories of travels in Spain." While not everybody waxes rhapsodic, they all have nice things to say, like "good paella, and a good Spanish guitarist on weekends."

FOOD ROOM STAFF COST

Taquet at the Wayne Hotel

$40

139 E. Lancaster Ave., Wayne (610) 687-5005
at Louella Ave. on the Main Line

While many Romac Reporters still consider this the "best French on the Main Line," enough dissenters say it's "not what it used to be" to drop its scores into the very good rather than the excellent range. Even those who think Jean-Francois Taquet is "the best saucier around" are inclined to note that portions are small. Those trying to hold down the cost opt for a prix fixe menu or eating in the lounge. The cruvinet provides 50 wines by the glass, one of the largest selections around.

Tavern, The

$23

261 Montgomery Ave., Bala Cynwyd (610) 664-3000
next to the firehouse on the Main Line

Here is an "old, reliable neighborhood" spot with an owner who is "always welcoming to the guests." The Traditional American food is also reliably good, with some of the more consistent numbers on our survey. There may be few surprises, but, sitting by the fire on a chilly winter evening, at a place that's called "a Main Line tradition," who wants surprises?

Tavern on Green

$20

2047 Green St., Philadelphia (215) 235-6767
at 21st St. in the Art Museum Area

Kemosabe say, Tavern on Green "best kept secret in town." Him say, "good beer," "best margarita." Him say, Tavern on Green have "wonderful atmosphere," good choice Art Museum area. Him wonder why name not "Tavern on the Green." Oh, it's on Green Street, that's why.

Tequila's

$25

1511 Locust St., Philadelphia (215) 546-0181
bet. 15th & 16th Sts. in Center City

"Don't let the exterior fool you," at this Center City Mexican, inside you'll find what is "arguably Philly's best Mexican food." The owner and chef are from Mexico City, and the food is just as authentic, though from all points South of the Border. With very good marks all around, the "tasty and potent drinks" stand out, as does "the best steak in the area, believe it or not." Ask for the waiters' help if you're not sure, they're "friendly and fun."

Tex Mex Connection/ Wales Junction Tavern

$20

Walnut & 2nd St, N. Wales (215) 699-9552
Sumneytown Pk. & North Wales Rd. in Montgomery County

Those who consider this spot by the North Wales train station "one of the best Tex-Mex eateries outside the Southwest" tend to think the "great gathering-place bar detracts from the dining experience." Those who think the bar serves "the best margaritas this side of Acapulco" beg to differ. Pastries are made in-house, the "decorations are well done," the "staff tries hard" and the restaurant offers children's specials. It's clear why the Connection is chugging into its second decade.

 = Superior = Excellent = Very Good

Thai Garden

$20

101 N. 11th St., Philadelphia (215) 629-9939 in Chinatown

"Creative, beautiful and innovative food, right in Chinatown" at this highly-rated Thai restaurant. Most voters call it "the best," and say the "dishes themselves are works of art." With a full page of vegetarian options, we hear it's even "nice enough for a special date." You might want to try the "best steamed dumplings this side of Thailand," or "any dish with fish."

Thai Pepper

$21

64 E. Lancaster Ave., Ardmore (610) 642-5951
Across from Lower Merion Twp. Bldg. on the Main Line

This little BYO in Ardmore has been getting lots of attention since it opened a little over two years ago. Most of our voters think the food is "very good," or even "excellent," saying that, at least "for the suburbs," they have "the best Thai around." With the kind of hype they've received from local press, however, some voters are bound to be disappointed, expecting a fancy slice of heaven and instead getting a tasty little BYO that offers takeout.

Thai Singha House

$18

3939 Chestnut St., Philadelphia (215) 382-8001
bet. 39th & 40th in University City/W. Phila.

Though it may be "expensive, compared with other Thais," most reviewers say it has the "most consistently delicious" "authentic" Thai food in Philadelphia. Its food rating is among the top in our polling area, and the "interesting menu" includes green curry chicken, flaming duck, and Thai iced tea.

Thomas'

$30

4201 Main St., Philadelphia (215) 483-9075
Main & Pensdale Sts. in Manayunk/Roxborough

What this Manayunk Continental/American lacks in service ("ordinary," say expectant voters) is easily made up for in the "great atmosphere," and might well be caused by it. You see, they have three floors here, with dining more formal as you go up, with a lovely balcony on the third floor, overlooking the second. Running up and down those stairs all night would bring even the most professional waiter to his knees. Fans say the food is "really good." Reservations essential.

Tierra

VOTE

100 Old Gulph Rd., Gulph Mills (610) 520-1200
at Upper Gulph Rd. in Montgomery County

The few Romac voters who have made it out to this Gulph Mills Mediterranean (since it opened in June) tell us that chef/owner Alan Segal makes it well worth the drive. Located on the same site as the old Picket Post, the setting is historic though the influences are now more Mediterranean than Colonial American. Combine it with the "excellent, imaginative food" and professional staff, and despite "high prices" we hear Tierra is "truly superb."

FOOD ROOM STAFF COST

Tiffany Dining Place & Gazebo

$23

799 DeKalb Pk., Centre Square (610) 275-4050
Rt. 202, just north of Rt. 73 in Montgomery County

You can eat until you turn Tiffany blue at this American dining place. It has an "excellent brunch, and you don't get rushed out," and the "ice cream sundae bar" is a favorite with the kids. Breakfasts, desserts and a "great salad bar" are standouts, with the rest of the menu only pulling down average marks.

Tira Misu

$37

528 S. 5th St., Philadelphia (215) 925-3335
bet. South & Lombard in the South St. Area

Named for the delightful Italian layered confection, of course Tira Misu specializes in dessert. Happily, everything before the dessert is also "outstanding." They serve Roman "Jewish-Italian" food that most call "delicious," and though service can be "strange," it doesn't seem to take away from their "professional" rating. We hear it's "worth every penny."

Toland's Wheel Pump

$21

529 Bethlehem Pk., Erdenheim (215) 836-9438
at Gordon Rd. in Montgomery County

"Decent pasta and seafood dishes, in a threadbare restaurant." That's what voters say about this Classic American Seafood restaurant in Erdenheim. Though the decor gets rapped, folks like the mural and say the bar upstairs is "very nice." "Casual and comfortable," reviewers say "solid food served in generous portions keeps this place very busy."

Tony Luke's

$10

39 E. Oregon Ave., Philadelphia (215) 551-5725
at Front St. in So. Phila.

While Tony Luke's technical food category is "American," we would suggest they change it to "Philadelphian." Not only are the cheesesteaks in the top 10, it's also in the top 10 for pre-game dining at the Vet and the Spectrum. A takeout spot, with sidewalk dining in nice weather, Tony Luke's (on an "interesting corner") is "more than just a cheesesteak:" "Uncle Mike's Sandwich is great for vegetarians," and "pork, aged provolone and greens, oh boy!"

Toscana Cucina Rustica

$33

24 N. Merion Ave., Bryn Mawr Mews, Bryn Mawr (610) 527-7700
at Lancaster Ave. on the Main Line

This "chic," bustling Main Line Italian specializes in the rustic food of Tuscany, and does it well enough to rank as "the finest Italian in the suburbs" for many voters. The open kitchen and wood-burning brick oven set a sophisticated tone. There's less agreement about the service; some praise it as "attentive," others—especially those likely to call the restaurant "overpriced"—criticize it as "haughty."

 = Superior = Excellent = Very Good

Totaro's

$35

729 E. Hector St., Conshohocken (610) 828-9341 in Montgomery County

With many wines by the glass, a staff that earns a "very good" rating, and of course "very good" food, it's no wonder that you have to "reserve weeks ahead" for this Conshohocken Italian. The "wonderful fresh entrees," while "interesting," may be "priced like one of Center City's finest," but the high ratings justify it. Don't be put off by the exterior: "You'd never know from the outside how good it is inside."

Trattoria San Nicola

VOTE

668 Lancaster Ave., Berwyn (610) 296-3141 on the Main Line

Though it opened after our polling deadline, we had to include this lovely little Berwyn Italian trattoria in the book, if not to recommend it, then to alert our participants to vote on it for next year's poll. With the same owners as Monte Carlo Living Room, both Primaveras and the Primavera Pizza Kitchen, this Main Line newcomer is one to watch.

Tree Tops at the Rittenhouse

$33

210 W. Rittenhouse Sq., Phila. (215) 790-2533 (19th St. in Ctr. City)

A "beautiful view" of Rittenhouse Square combines with "conservatory decor" to make the room and ambiance the big winner at this Center City American. It was close, though; very good food and staff ratings help put Tree Tops on the list of Philly's favorites. We hear it has the "best ladies' business lunch," "good weekend brunches" and Christmas and New Years' dinners, and "fun twilight specials" that offer an economical look at one of the top views in the city.

Tre Scalini

VOTE

1533 S. 11th St., Phila. (215) 551-3870 (at Tasker in So. Phila.)

This two-year-old South Philly spot features the food of central Italy, and the voters who have discovered it say it serves "good food at reasonable prices." The turn-off for Romac Reporters is the room—"Why is the lighting so bright?" one asks.

Triangle Tavern

$18

10th & Reed Sts., Philadelphia (215) 467-8683 in So. Phila.

This South Philly Italian is over 50 and remains popular despite food ratings that are only fair—and the room and staff score even lower. But the beloved dive is "fun and funky," "memorable for entertainment, mussels and pizza." Stop in for "spaghetti before Flyers games" and you, too, might find "this place brings back nothing but good memories." N.B. park across the street at the Acme.

Trieste

VOTE

641 Chester Pk., Prospect Park (610) 534-8191 at Rt. 420 in Delaware County

A few voters have stumbled upon this Southern Italian in Prospect Park. Maybe it's for the "very good" food, and "lots of it," but we're betting it also has something to do with the fact that it's "good for families." Reasonably priced, Trieste also has a dozen wines by the glass.

FOOD ROOM STAFF COST

Trolley Stop

$25

4043 Skippack Pk., Skippack (610) 584-4849
Valley Forge Rd. & Rt. 363 in Montgomery County

In their efforts to make this American and Italian Seafood and Steakhouse (car?) a train-based dining experience the chef/owner may have gone too far. Voters complain that it's "loud," with only so-so food, at least at dinner. Still, with "great brussell sprouts" and "good early bird specials," at moderate prices, it's a good stop for lunch or a bite before prime-time.

Tsui Hang Chun

VOTE

911 Race St., Philadelphia (215) 925-8901
betw. 9th. & 10th. in Chinatown

While not too many folks know about this very authentic Chinese, those who do say it is very good. With typical Chinatown features, like Chinese music in the background, dim sum early in the day, and what seems like preferential treatment to Asian customers, we're hoping this two-year-old gets more traffic and makes our voters feel more welcome.

Turf Club

$17

1635 Market St., Philadelphia (215) 246-1556
17th & Market in Center City

It's a good bet none of your fellow diners stopped by Philadelphia Park's off-track betting parlor just for the food. The menu is basic and pitched more to the $2 bettors than the high-stakes players—steak for the winners, hamburgers for those who are ripping up their tickets.

Tutto Misto

$28

603 S. 3rd St., Philadelphia (215) 923-7220
at South St. in the South St. Area

This new South Street area spot is a mixed bag—downstairs a tapas bar and bistro seven days a week with lunch on weekends, upstairs a Mediterranean dining room with fixed-price dinners Wednesdays through Saturdays. The food scores show an odd split—many say average, almost as many say excellent, few say very good. The tapas generally get better grades; the upstairs room is more often called "a lovely place without food to match."

12th Street Cantina

$9

45 N. 12th St., Reading Terminal Market, Philadelphia
(215) 625-0321 bet. Market & Arch in Center City

This Reading Terminal Market stall is popular both for its classic Mexican fare, and for modern dishes like lamb in orange adobe sauce and pork with roasted tomato salsa. Patrons can eat in until 4 or take it out until 6.

 = **Superior** = **Excellent** = **Very Good**

Umbria

$30

7131 Germantown Ave., Philadelphia (215) 242-6470 at Mt. Airy in Chestnut Hill/Mt. Airy

A "lovely little haven," this Chestnut Hill Eclectic (focusing mainly on Italian and Continental dishes) has a big group of fans for such a small (42 seat) restaurant. Called "a hidden gem," it's one of those places our voters ask us to keep under wraps. They also think Umbria should change their menu more often, while rejoicing that this BYO is just down the block from the State Store.

Under the Blue Moon

$31

8042 Germantown Ave., Philadelphia (215) 247-1100 at Abington Ave. in Chestnut Hill/Mt. Airy

What makes this International Eclectic and American restaurant one of Philly's favorites? Some try to analyze it, calling the food "very good," the atmosphere "congenial, interesting, even romantic." More bluntly, one voter says it's "just fun—and good food." It's always crowded, and the owner, Gene Gosfield, is "still crazy after all these years." Worth a look, for the "only unstuffy place in Chestnut Hill."

Upstares at Varalli

$26

1345 Locust St., Philadelphia (215) 546-4200 at Broad St. in Center City

Though the name's a bit flighty, the Northern Italian cooking is very good at this very popular Center City spot, which boasts an excellent view of the Academy of Music. "A great place to go before the orchestra," or even after the theater, reserve ahead, because there's a line out the door for the "fantastic bread," pre-theater specials, and what one diner calls "the best Caesar I've had." Room and staff also do well, and for all that, the price makes it a good value.

U.S. Hotel Bar & Grill

$25

4439 Main St., Philadelphia (215) 483-9222 at Green Ln.. in Manayunk/Roxborough

This "New Orleans-style" bar ("fun in the afternoons" is part of that scene) is full of "lots of friendly Manayunk locals," being served by what one voters calls the "best bartenders." Sundays and Thursdays, there are "great little bands" performing live, but unfortunately the kitchen does not win such mass appeal: the food is only "so-so," and "overly expensive" to some voters.

Valley Green Inn

$28

Springfield Ave. & Wissahickon Creek, Philadelphia (215) 247-1730 in Chestnut Hill/Mt. Airy

"The setting is the real winner" at this country inn, from the "great ambiance" of the room to the "charming and peaceful" views of Fairmount Park, "a good place to walk off dinner." No matter how "romantic" the setting, the food disappoints our voters. Though the menu is unimaginative, we hear the Valley Green is a "good place to take your folks."

FOOD ROOM STAFF COST

Valley Stream Inn

$32

748 Bridgetown Pk., Langhorne (215) 750-1994
at Street Rd. in Bucks County

Most of the votes hit the "very good" mark at this Langhorne American, with a few naysayers pulling the averages down because of an off evening or two. The views of the creek and woods are nice, the nightly live piano entertaining and the homemade desserts are favorites, and the great "breakfast and brunch buffets," particularly on holidays, stand out as "inexpensive and tasty."

Vang Garden (fka Van's Garden)

$13

121 N. 11th St., Philadelphia (215) 923-2438
bet. Race & Arch in Chinatown

While there are better Vietnamese restaurants in Chinatown and elsewhere, there are few cheaper. That's not the only reason to recommend this little place, according to our voters. The food can be "very good," and the service "charming." "Love that Vietnamese coffee!"

Vickers Tavern

$39

192 E. Welsh Pool Rd., Lionville (610) 363-7998
at Gordon Dr. in Chester County

Once a stop on the Underground Railroad, this historic Continental located in a farmhouse in Lionville has "consistently fine food" and an "excellent" setting. Nearly everyone agrees that the "high-quality gourmet entrees," though perhaps a bit "old-fashioned," are "worth the price." This is a special spot, so you'll probably feel more comfortable dressing up. In winter, "sit by the fire and enjoy a wonderful meal," or dine outside in warmer weather.

Victor Cafe

$33

1303 Dickenson St., Philadelphia (215) 468-3040
at 13th St. in So. Phila.

Food ratings remain steady, but ambiance and staff ratings couldn't get any higher at this South Philly Northern Italian. Of course, we think that has to do with the "great singing waiters," whose "wonderful entertainment" makes this place a "must for visitors from out of town." But what is "charming" to some is an "overpriced tourist trap" to others. One regular of 35 years sums it up: "The food is fair, it's just fun!"

Vietnam

$16

221 N. 11th St., Philadelphia (215) 592-1163
bet. Race & Vine Sts. in Chinatown

Despite "plastic table cloths and all," this unassuming and inexpensive Vietnamese restaurant in Chinatown has made it into the top 40 for food in our poll. "Kind and efficient waiters" serve "authentic," "excellent," even "amazingly outstanding" food, and most agree it's "inexpensive, and better and healthier than Chinese food." Though the ambiance is "lousy," it is also "very clean."

 = Superior = Excellent = Very Good

Vietnam Palace

$15

222 N. 11 St., Philadelphia (215) 592-9596
bet. Race & Vine Sts. in Chinatown

You won't find any fancy-pants French influences at this "wonderful," very authentic Vietnamese restaurant in Chinatown. Family owned and run, they specialize in beef dishes, including one order called "seven courses of beef." One somewhat alarmed reviewer notes that, like other Chinatown spots, "they have one room for Asians, one for non-Asians."

Villa Di Roma

$21

936 S. 9th St., Philadelphia (215) 592-1295
bet. Washington & Christian Sts. in So. Phila.

This old-fashioned South Philly Italian "tradition" has "the best mussels anywhere," and its location, amid the Italian Market, ensures freshness. Regulars laud the consistency and tout the Chicken Neapolitan and Veal Sicilian; less frequent patrons claim the staff "cater to their 'own' customers."

Village Cafe

VOTE

Hollow & Flowing Spring Rds., Birchrunville (610) 827-0930
in Chester County

Everything is homemade at this Chesco Country Cafe, and it's "food beyond compare in the middle of nowhere." Our voters call the food "gourmet, and imaginative," and the "high quality" is "consistent." You must reserve—the room only seats 40—and it has many fans who keep going back. Be warned: "Crossing the outdoor porch to get to the bathroom in winter can be a bummer."

Village Porch Bistro

$19

Olde Sproul Village, Springfield (610) 544-3220
Baltimore Pk. & Rt. 320 in Delaware County

The more vocal Romac Reporters consistently call this Delaware County Modern American in Olde Sproul Village "a great surprise" and wonder, "How can a former ice cream parlor be this good?" Most rave about the "interesting ingredient combinations" and "great sandwiches" on a menu that changes weekly while praising the casual yet "quaint" Victorian room, filled with "antiques galore." The ice cream is still top-notch, too. The restaurant is dry, though, so remember to bring your own wine.

Villanova Diner

$13

797 E. Lancaster Ave., Villanova (610) 527-9009
Rts. 320 & 30 on the Main Line

This Greek Diner in Villanova may have low ratings, but it does have one thing going for it: It's right off Rt. 476. One thrifty eater calls it "the poor man's power breakfast."

FOOD ROOM STAFF COST

Villa Rosa

$18

661 Heacock Rd., Edgewood Shopping Ctr., Yardley
(215) 321-0850 in Bucks County

Despite "no ambiance," the "lines of people waiting stretch out the door" at this "strip-mall Italian" in Yardley. We suspect it has more to do with the low prices than the "basic food."

Villa Strafford

$43

115 Strafford Ave., Wayne (610) 964-1116
at Lancaster Ave. on the Main Line

The votes are in on this Wayne American/International, and it's a winner. Set in a restored colonial mansion, many consider it one of "the Main Line's best." With an Italian owner taking care of the management, and a German chef taking care of the kitchen, it just misses the favorites list because some think it's a bit "stuffy." Closed on Sunday, and reservations are essential.

Vincent's

$31

1373 Easton Rd., Warrington (215) 343-0210
Bristol Rd. & 611 in Bucks County

This is the kind of historic-setting, Italian and Continental spot where they prepare the Caesar salad at your tableside, are smoker friendly, and let dinner unfold at a leisurely pace. But, ten years in Warrington have seen the prices climb, while the menu has remained relatively unchanged. To get the most out of this place, try the early bird specials, or go on weekends when the piano player is there.

Vincent's

$27

10 E. Gay St., West Chester (610) 696-4262 (High St. in Chester Cty.)

The Continental food at this West Chester spot is "solid, often surprising." But while "the menu doesn't seem to change much," neither does the sound provided by jazz pianist Al Russell on weekends (a quartet plays on Thursdays). If you're up for this "suave excursion for dinner," reservations are essential.

Vinh Hoa

$20

746 Christian St., Phila. (215) 925-0307 (8th & Christian in S. Phila.)

Though this South Philly spot is not popular with Romac Reporters, it is one of the few Vietnamese/Chinese restaurants in the area, and one of the only places where our voters can sample ingredients like lemon grass and cinnamon leaves. Once Vinh Hoa gets more attention, we think it will become a contender.

Vitale's

$22

2100 St. Vincent St., Phila. (215) 624-5015
Cottman & Bustleton Aves. in Northeast Phila.

Patrick Vitale took over for his father, and has kept the great Italian American tradition of this Northeast Philly spot very much alive. With "great food and service at a great price," this local bar and restaurant only gets bad marks for the somewhat iffy decor. There's lots to choose from, with a kids' menu and fifteen wines by the glass.

 = Superior = Excellent = Very Good

Volare

$27

4421 Main St., Philadelphia (215) 483-9797 in Manayunk/Roxborough

With the same owners as South Philly's Cafe Longano, a few are calling this Regional Italian that area's "best new restaurant." With cozy, hand painted "incredible decor," and "very good food" in "good-sized portions," early reports say that they're still working out those new restaurant kinks: service can be "inattentive," and the reservation policy doesn't mean you won't have to wait. But our voters are sure this "very welcoming" spot "will improve with age."

Waldorf Cafe

$26

20th & Lombard Sts., Philadelphia (215) 985-1836 in Center City

This little American bistro, located in Center City, has a loyal following, though some one-or-two-time diners left unimpressed. It is kid-friendly and unassuming, and mid-priced for what one fan calls "food cooked to perfection."

Walt's

$19

806 S. 2nd St., Phila. (215) 339-9124 at Catherine St. in So. Phila.

The Queen Village Seafood spot is one of the city's best-loved dives, and also is the No. 2 crabhouse. The kitchen and menu have been expanded, but fans go for the old-fashioned seafood dishes. One voter sums it up: "good food, low prices, no atmosphere, cash only."

Warmdaddy's Blues

VOTE

Front & Market Sts., Philadelphia (215) 627-2500 in the Historic Area

This brand-new southern cuisine and blues club opened on Front and Market Street too recently for many of our voters to get a bead on it: early reports say it might be the first place to successfully combine "excellent live blues" with "great food." Why don't y'all give it a try, sugah?

Warsaw Cafe

$26

306 S. 16th St., Philadelphia (215) 546-0204 at Spruce St. in Center City

While this Center City place has many fans, we suspect that the naysayers, who bring the ratings down to just "good", didn't know what to expect from the Central and Eastern European menu. From seafood kugels to hot and cold borscht, lamb stew and fish entrees that make up the "interesting menu," this "small, intimate place" is worth a visit.

Water Wheel

VOTE

1526 Sansom St., Philadelphia (215) 563-9601 bet. 15th & 16th in Center City

The owner's of Jonathon's have added a location at the site of an old favorite—Charlie's Water Wheel. Too new for our participants to vote on, we refer you to the Jonathon's deli review, and note that this is one of the few kosher places in town.

FOOD ROOM STAFF COST

West End Saloon

$21

State & Orange Sts., Media (610) 566-3260 in Delaware County

Some folks recommend this neighborhood Italian in Media for weekday lunch: that's one clue that what they do here are the simpler things. But what they do best is for the after work crowd, with great bartenders and waitresses, and plenty of amusements like pool tables, tabletop shuffleboard and a big screen TV.

Westgate Pub

$17

1021 W. Chester Pk., Havertown (610) 446-3030
at Manoa Rd. in Delaware County

For "great casual dining" with a "big, varied menu," stop in at this Delco Italian-American. It's "a great family restaurant" with low prices and "big portions," so it sometimes gets "crowded and noisy" and "too smoky."

West Point Tavern (fka Johan's)

VOTE

West Point Pk. & Garfield Ave., West Point (215) 699-3352
in Montgomery County

As far from the mess hall as you can get is this American Tavern, recently reopened by the same management as City Tavern after a renovation (to a Civil War/turn-of-the-century theme) and name change. The "great menu" has lots of options, maybe too many: It "even has sweetbreads on it." There's also a place for pipe and cigar smokers, and a great Sunday brunch buffet.

White Dog Cafe

$29

3420 Sansom St., Philadelphia (215) 386-9224
bet. 34th & 36th in University City/W. Phila.

You'll find this University City favorite all over our "Tops by" section in the front of the book, with conversation, brunch and bar food as standouts among the lists. It's also ranked third in Philadelphian's favorites, most likely for the "generous portions" of "new age" food, including "fabulous rolls and breads." "There's always something new to try," but a few are frustrated by the huge crowds, long reservation lead-times, and sometimes "too politically correct" atmosphere.

Whitemarsh Valley Inn

$29

474 Germantown Pk., Lafayette Hill (610) 941-0555
at Joshua Road in Montgomery County

The oak interior, piano background music and beef-heavy menu give this Montgomery County Continental an old-fashioned ambiance. Some say it's "a little expensive for a suburban family restaurant."

Wildflowers

$16

8 N Mechanic St., New Hope (215) 862-2241
at Main St. in Bucks County

This American with Mexican touches occupies the oldest building in New Hope and overlooks Ingham Creek, making it a "great romantic place to eat," a "cheerful lunch place with some vegetarian specialties." Regulars say the food is "good but uneven," and "the room upstairs is the best" place to enjoy it.

Wild Onion

$24

900 Conestoga Rd., Rosemont (610) 527-4826 (Garrett Ave., Main Line)

This Main Line Regional American centers around its bar, but many voters, especially younger ones, say it has "good food at good prices." Some like the menu's more creative efforts like the Shrimp Napoleon, others praise the "delicious beef stew" and "garlicky mashed potatoes." The main complaint: "One time it's fantastic, the next disappointing," and the staff is "so young they don't quite understand good service."

William Penn Inn

$32

Rt. 202 & Sumneytown Pk., Gwynedd (215) 699-9272 (Montgomery Cty.)

Old Bill would be proud that his name was used for such an "excellent" spot in Montgomery County. On our Top 10 list for brunch, it's very high on our list of Philadelphian's favorites. "Last of the 'inn-style' restaurants, the William Penn is worth a trip," especially for the "early bird soup or salad, with great desserts."

Williamson Restaurant

$26

Belmont & City Aves., Atop the GSB Building, Bala Cynwyd (215) 839-7946 (in the City Line Area)

This City Line area American restaurant is a favorite among older diners. Perhaps the "great view," from the top of the GSB Building is what brings them in. More likely it is the "wonderful" staff, that "goes out of its way," that has made this "a favorite" for 50 years.

Willistown Grille

$28

4 Manor Rd., Paoli (610) 695-8990 (off Lancaster Ave. on the Main Line)

This Northern Italian/Provincial French restaurant in Paoli was recently remodeled, and our voters think the food is improving, too. The charming room is notable for the large, two-way fireplace that opens onto both the dining room and the bar. Light and airy in the day, the linen tablecloths, candles and flowers add to the romantic atmosphere at night.

Wycombe Inn

$40

1073 Mill Creek Rd., Wycombe (215) 598-7000
1 mile west of Rt. 413 in Bucks County

The American-Continental cuisine and English pub atmosphere fit right into the historic village of Wycombe, creating a restaurant voters "really enjoy." Older reporters appreciate the ambiance, particularly the piano music in the bar on weekends. Also offers Sunday brunch.

Yangming

$30

1051 Conestoga Rd., Bryn Mawr (610) 527-3200
at Haverford Rd. on the Main Line

Great food, and a "high-class atmosphere" have put this Main Line Chinese restaurant in the Top 100 for food and popularity—though it might be "too popular." Either way, a throng of diners agree that it might be the "best Chinese in the 'burbs," if a little pricey. But you get a lot for your dollar, in service and in "lovely atmosphere." In short, "a beautiful restaurant, and not your typical Chinese food."

FOOD ROOM STAFF COST

Yellow Springs, Inn at Historic

$37

Art School Rd., Chester Springs (610) 827-7477
Near Rts. 113 & 401 in Chester County

Not just another superb French Continental historic country inn, for while the food and staff are rated "very good," the setting is characterized as "idyllic." The Inn seems to cater to an older crowd, with most of the votes coming from the over-40's. One incurable romantic offers that it's "a great date night with your wife."

Ye Olde Ale House

$16

405 E. Germantown Pk., Lafayette Hill (610) 825-2469
Joshua Rd. & Germantown Pk. in Montgomery County

Hand carved roast beef sandwiches, roast pork and hot wings make up the Tavern menu at this 25-year-old Lafayette hill spot. "The roast beef sandwiches are out of this world" according to voters, who are also fans of the low price tag.

Ye Olde Temperance House

$36

5-11 S. State St., Newtown (215) 860-0474 in Bucks County

While our voters say "the food is so-so," they advise that it "can be great if you hit a night with good specials." But while the food may sometimes miss, the "great jazz music" is always a hit. Call ahead for a schedule of events, and don't worry about bringing that bathtub gin—the Temperance may be Olde, but the liquor license is definitely newe.

Yorktown Inn

$25

8121 Old York Rd., Yorktown Courtyard & Shoppes, Elkins Park (215) 887-0600 at Church Rd. in Montgomery County

This Montgomery County Continental, opened in 1957 and rebuilt after a fire in 1989, sticks to traditional fare in an early American, fairly dressy atmosphere (jackets are requested).

Zanzibar Blue

$32

305 S. 11th St., Philadelphia (215) 829-0300
bet. Spruce & Pine Sts. in Center City

"Still the best Jazz bar in Philadelphia," Romac Reviewers voted this upscale International restaurant-cum-jazz club number one for Live Entertainment in our poll. Good any night, the Sunday jazz brunch stands out as a highlight. With "novel and interesting" Caribbean specialties, the wine list is a Romac Top 10. "The people," say voters, "make the place."

Zocalo

$29

3600 Lancaster Ave., Philadelphia (215) 895-0139
1 blk. north of Market St. in University City/W. Phila.

In Mexico City, the Zocalo is the center of town, and in the Delaware Valley, Zocalo is the center of the Contemporary Mexican food universe. "Their outdoor tables are charming," and you might need that fresh air after tasting the highly-recommended "Hotter than Hell shrimp." While the waitstaff could use a swift kick in the serape, this place may well be "the best Mexican in town."

 = Superior = Excellent = Very Good

New Jersey

Acacia

$44

2637 Main St., Lawrenceville (609) 895-9885
at Franklin Corner Rd. in Central Jersey

"This is the place to go" for "wonderful, creative" contemporary American food, "elegant" atmosphere, and "great" service, that is. Crafted from an old post office, this "lovely" little spot may be "pricey" (though you can BYO), but it's certainly "worth a trip" for chef-owner Bryan Brodowski's terrific, seasonally changing food, which helped garner Acacia Top Overall ratings in the state. "Great for business dinners," even though it's out in the country.

Adelphia

$20

1796 Clements-Bridge Rd., Deptford (609) 845-8200
at Rt. 42 in So. Jersey

The Deptford wives (and husbands) don't know it, but this big, Victorian-style Continental serves decent if unsurprising food, in particular a prix fixe dinner-for-two at $19.95. Daily early birds are another gold mine, and there's a pretty terrace when the weather's fine. Good luck finding better bargains for atmosphere like this, anywhere.

Alchemist & Barrister

$31

28 Witherspoon St., Princeton (609) 924-5555
at Nassau St. in Central Jersey

Voters say this pubby American is "the only place in Princeton for education and culture." The "versatile," moderately priced menu features something for everyone, from burgers and sandwiches to full-scale dinners, and there's pub grub until midnight for late-night sustenance. These comfortable, well-aged quarters are chockablock with students, locals, tourists—making this one of the town's "favorites." It's "good for brunch," especially when the pretty patio is in use.

Alexander's Inn

$35

653 Washington St., Cape May (609) 884-2555
bet. Ocean & Franklin at the Jersey Shore

If this teeny Cape May French proves one thing, it's that bigger isn't necessarily better. Most voters give the historic Victorian setting the very top marks, with the attentive, professional staff and "very good" food running a close second and third. Everything, from appetizers to desserts, is made on the premises, a "romantic, delicious" meal that's "appetizing for all the senses."

Al Kimah

$25

1426 Rt. 70 E., Pinetree Plaza, Cherry Hill (609) 427-0888 in So. Jersey

"The more the merrier" at this "very unique" Moroccan, with its inexpensive, multi-course menu, Lawrence of Arabia ambience, and "very sensual" belly dancers. You feel like you're dining in a Berber tent, complete with comfortable low couches, brass tables, and hand-washing between courses. It attracts a young, sometimes boisterous crowd (full-size coolers for BYO sometimes spotted), but the "exotic" food is authentic enough (bastilla, tajines, and so on) to please aficionados too. All in all, "a fun night for everyone."

FOOD ROOM STAFF COST

Angeloni's II

$29

2400 Arctic Ave., Atlantic City (609) 344-7875
at Georgia Ave. at the Jersey Shore
Family-owned and authentic-tasting, this atmospheric old-line Ducktown Italian-American attracts a largely local crowd who like the extensive, traditional menu (seafood and hand-cut steaks a specialty) and a surprising wine list that's good enough to catch a Wine Spectator award. Though it doesn't seem to have caught on with our Reporters yet, this is a great alternative to the overpriced casino joints.

Angelo's Fairmount Tavern

$28

2300 Fairmount Ave., Atlantic City (609) 344-2439
at Mississippi Ave. at the Jersey Shore
"Huge portions" of "good food" (subset: red-sauce Italian) are the reason many traditionalists "won't go to another restaurant at the Shore." The Thirties-era ambiance may be "basic" and the service only fair, but this family-owned and -operated A.C. mainstay hasn't been in business for 60 years for nothing.

Arizona

$20

801 N. Blackhorse Pk., Runnemeade (609) 939-2263 (So. Jersey)
Well, not exactly, but it's as close to the southwest as you can get at this "very casual," "fresh" and "friendly" little place that mixes it up with Italian and "Tex-Mex" favorites. Prices are rock-bottom, including two daily $14.95 specials. BYO keeps checks lower still.

Athens Cafe

$19

1030 Rt. 70 W., Cherry Hill (609) 429-1061
at Cooper Landing Rd. in So. Jersey
Friendly and relaxed, this little-known Greek BYO offers the only non-diner Greek cooking in South Jersey, including homestyle specialties like moussaka and stuffed grape-vine leaves. Sure, it's "not Dmitri's," but this atmospheric cafe is a whole lot closer—and less crowded.

Axelsson's Blue Claw

VOTE

991 Ocean Dr., Cape May (609) 884-5878 (at the Jersey Shore)
"Best seafood on the Shore" say fans of this Cape May staple that specializes in—of course—crab cakes and "great clam dishes." Water views and "great prices" belie the "refreshingly elegant" European-style decor, complete with tablecloths, fresh flowers and piano music wafting from the more casual Clipper Ship Pub, all done up in cherry paneling. Dining in the outdoor garden in season ain't bad, either.

Back Yard

$34

220 81st St., Stone Harbor (609) 368-2627
at Dune Dr. at the Jersey Shore
This teeny Stone Harbor French (that also serves a smattering of Northern Italian dishes) more than doubles in size when they have outdoor dining avalailable. Even so, be sure you "definitely eat outdoors—and make reservations!" For great soft shell crabs on a cool summer night, some say it's the "best dining experience at the shore."

 = Superior = Excellent = Very Good

Barnacle Ben's

$20

Kings Hwy. & Lenola Rd., Kingsway Plaza, Maple Shade (609) 235-5808 (in So. Jersey)

The "freshest seafood, well prepared" more than compensates for the "tacky" shopping-mall-nautical decor at this wildly popular storefront at an equally busy intersection in Maple Shade. Cognoscenti recommend the crab au gratin ("the best") and the seafood salad ("loaded" with shrimp and so on), but there's also 16 different types of finny fish, and you can raid your own wine cellar before you come to wait on line.

Beau Rivage

$43

128 Taunton Blvd., Medford (609) 983-1999 at Tuckerton Rd. in So. Jersey

"A four-star place in the woods" pretty much sums up the sentiment on this dressy (don't forget that tie!), "sophisticated" Provincial French standby. Though "consistency can be a problem at times," most of reviewers laud the "romantic" setting, "refined" service, and "excellent food." "Enchanting gardens" overlooking Lake Pine and a superior wine list add to the "charming" experience. Pricey, yes, but you'll like it, too.

Benihana

$35

5255 Marlton Pk., Pennsauken (609) 665-6320 bet. 38 & 70 in So. Jersey

Good food becomes "great entertainment" right at your tableside, at this much imitated Japanese chop shop chain. Watch your chef wield that cutlery, he's a bad mother—but don't shut your mouth, open it up to great teppan yaki and steaks, among other fresh Japanese specialties. "A great place for a special event," we hear, "or to impress your friends."

Braddock's Tavern

$34

39 S. Main St., Medford Village (609) 654-1604 at Coates St. in So. Jersey

"Perfect for business and romance" is this "old-style tavern experience" in the pretty little town of Medford Village. Located in a beautifully restored 19th-century building, Braddock's is "nice for special occasions," "family celebrations," or anytime you want to soak up "delightful" "Colonial ambiance" (candlelight, fireplaces, and wide-plank floors) and well-regarded "early American food" (game and crab cakes are specialties). It's "sort of expensive," but all in all, "a wonderful way to dine out."

Brighton Steakhouse

$45

Brighton Park & Boardwalk, Sands Hotel & Casino, Atlantic City (609) 441-4300 (at the Jersey Shore)

When nothing else but double Porterhouse will do, you could do worse than this good-looking steak specialist in the Sands Hotel & Casino—there's veal, lamb chops, and something called lobster popcorn, too. Live piano, an extravagant Sunday brunch buffet, and heads-up service are added enticements—and well they should be at these prices.

= Good = Fair [no rating] = Poor

FOOD ROOM STAFF COST

Brittany's Cafe

$25

4313 Ventnor Ave., Atlantic City (609) 348-8741
at DeLancey Pl. at the Jersey Shore

The poor decor at this tiny Atlantic City Italian restaurant, specializing in fish dishes, can be misleading. What they do well, they do the "best in the area," from omelettes in the morning, good lunches until 3 p.m., and "consistently" good dinner. The "excellent" service makes Brittany's a good bet; few seats make reservations a must.

Busch's

$34

8700 Landis Ave., Sea Isle City (609) 263-8626
at Pleasure St. at the Jersey Shore

"Generic seafood," yes, but locals flock to this no-nonsense spot that's been around—and in the same family—for over 100 years. The straightforward, reasonably priced food (deviled crab a specialty) is "adequate" but the ambiance is "fun"—"too bad" the "best she-crab" soup around is only available on Sunday and Tuesday. Closed mid-September to mid-May.

Caffe Aldo Lamberti

$28

2011 Rt. 70 W., Race Track Intersection, Cherry Hill
(609) 663-1747
at Haddonfield Rd. in So. Jersey

"Seen one, you've seen 'em all"—the Lamberti empire, that is, with its "awesome" service and elegant atmosphere, and classic Italian food that's "always good." For the record, this one's hard by the Garden State race track, and with all that implies, perhaps that's why prices are on the highish side compared with other Lamberti's.

Cafe Anecia

$20

414 Pavillion Ave., Riverside (609) 764-1155
at River Rd. in So. Jersey

In its fifth year, this Italian restaurant has really come into its own, according to our voters. Chef/owner Craig Quinlan cooks "very good" food to order, and keeps the prices reasonable. He has an "excellent" staff that's also very kid-friendly: In addition to welcoming parents with infants, there is a kid's menu and a toy box, plus crayons and paper, for the little ones.

Cafe Gallery

$37

219 High St., Burlington (609) 386-6150
at Pearl St. in So. Jersey

"Quality all around" characterizes this charming French-Continental cafe-cum-art gallery, locally lauded for its stupendous Sunday brunch buffet—"the best in the area." Artwork on the walls and a gorgeous view of the Delaware make for a "great setting" for "delightful" food. There's also a pretty riverfront garden terrace for outdoor dining when the weather's fine. No wonder it's sometimes tough to get a reservation.

= Superior = Excellent = Very Good

Cafe Loren

23rd & Dune Dr., Avalon (609) 967-8228 (at the Jersey Shore)
With only a handful of votes to go on, we hear that this pricey little Continental spot in Avalon is simply great. In summer, especially on weekends, you have to remember to call ahead, and don't forget to BYO. A good value for a "great meal."

Caffe LaBella

$27

61 E. Main St., Moorestown (609) 234-7755 (Chester Ave. in So. Jersey)
"Good Italian" and cozy atmosphere are the stock-in-trade of this little BYO cafe, located in a romantic circa-1685 building in historic Moorestown. Weekend breakfast, Sunday brunch, and an evening harpist make this a favorite of locals—if little-known by our surveyors. P.S. Cioppino is a house specialty.

Caffe La Bucca

$22

561 Haddonfield-Berlin Rd., 561 Plaza, Voorhees (609) 767-2250 at S. Gate Dr. in So. Jersey
In the same location as Mrs. London's used to be, this Italian restaurant in Voorhees, with a progressive menu, has quickly earned the reputation as a "terrific little neighborhood gourmet." With seating very limited, you must remember to reserve in advance, but it is worth it for the cozy, Italian/American ambiance, very friendly and professional staff, and even occasional live entertainment. BYO.

Camelot at Merv Griffin's

$34

1133 Boardwalk, Atlantic City (609) 344-6000 at N. Carolina Ave. at the Jersey Shore
Hoo, boy. Camelot is the theme at this pricey, high-concept steak-and-seafood joint, all tripped out like a medieval banquet hall with costumed minstrels, heavy drapes and big, private chairs where you can be naughty and never seen. The food at this "terrific" casino restaurant is judged very good and the service, "outstanding," so get out of the nineties, and give it a try. Extra points for the salad bar and "seafood feast."

Campbell's Seafood

$18

3231 Asbury Ave., Ocean City (609) 399-4337 (at the Jersey Shor)
Old-line American seafood on the cheap (heavy on the fried clams and shrimp, natch) is the stock-in-trade of this Ocean City standby, which has been serving takeout-food only to a generation of loyalists. The menu hasn't changed in decades (neither has the decor), but who cares when that means you can still get "the best" crab Imperial around? Closed October through April.

Capriccio at Merv Griffin's

$42

1133 Boardwalk, Merv Griffin's Resorts Casino Hotel, Atlantic City (609) 340-6457 (at the Jersey Shore)
Take your favorite person to listen to the strolling guitarist at this pricey formal casino Italian. "Ask for an ocean view table" at what some believe is "the best restaurant at the shore."

FOOD ROOM STAFF COST

Capuano

$19

806 Haddonfield Rd., Cherry Hill (609) 663-9119
at Race Track Cir. in So. Jersey

"A super place to BYOB and mange," this comfortable, pretty Mediterranean cafe prides itself on affordable, high-quality Italian food and gracious yet low-key service. Though not well-known outside the neighborhood, it attracts a loyal clientele who would like to keep its charms to themselves.

Catelli's

VOTE

Plaza 1000 Main St., Voorhees (609) 751-6069
in So. Jersey

This Voorhees Italian is newly opened, but has already acquired a following. During the holiday season, they have live entertainment, and during the nicer weather, they have dining on the patio. The food is "delicious," and the varied menu has imagination, with very special specials. "Not that noisy," notes one fan of conversation.

Charlie's Tavern

$20

800 Shore Rd., Somers Point (609) 927-3663
at New Jersey Ave. at the Jersey Shore

"Casual dining" and "excellent" chicken wings are the draw at this "beer-and-wings sports bar" that also serves moderately priced German and American-style tavern fare. The decor may be nothing more than TV sets and a pool table, but the staff is "exceptionally friendly" and Octoberfest in the parking lot is a Somers Point tradition. Extra bonus points for the late-night bar menu, but the credit-card-free policy may be a problem.

Chateau Silvana

$35

324 Main St., Medford (609) 654-1706
in So. Jersey

Tranquility, thy name is Silvana, courtesy of chef-owner Anthony Bonfiglio's beautiful 18th-century Georgian countryside farmhouse, lovingly restored as a candlelit, French/Italian inn. Though a few of our reporters grouse about "small portions for the price" and the ambitious food can be hit-or-miss, for most this gorgeous spot provides an experience "so pleasant sitting in a charming old inn watching horses jump in the fields outside."

Chef Vola

$33

111 S. Albion Pl., Atlantic City (609) 345-2022
at the Jersey Shore

Now that you have the number (it's not in the phone book), you still won't get a table at Chef Vola. How can this be? The food scores are just "good," the room is "noisy and crowded," and those punctured tomato cans, lit with light bulbs, ain't no Tiffanys. Moreover, the "tough time getting on the reservations list" makes our voters crabby. The charm is probably that it's family-owned and -operated, with a clientele who've been visiting for years. No credit cards.

Chianti's

701 Whittaker Ave., Trenton (609) 695-0011
at Beatty St. in Central Jersey

The medium size and moderate prices match the middle-of-the-road room at this otherwise "excellent Italian," located in Trenton. Decorated like an old Italian Tuscan villa, this Chambersburg area spot is a "local favorite," serving "great salads and desserts," with many heart-healthy options. They get quite busy on weekends, so be sure to call ahead.

Chili's

$16

1800 Clements Bridge Rd., Deptford (609) 384-1212
in S. Jersey
1310 Rt. 73 S., Mt. Laurel (609) 273-0020
in S. Jersey

Chili's scores look unimpressive until they're stacked up against similar chains. While some voters have had "awful" experiences, many say it's "a great place to take the kids—$1 per!" The food isn't great, but it's "better than you'd expect," and "children and parents can both enjoy it and be comfortable."

C.J. Muffin

$25

64 High St., Mt. Holly (609) 267-0025
at Beverley Rancocas Rd. in So. Jersey

Located in an old 1810 house, this locally popular, cutely named and trendy-menued spot (steak, seafood, Cajun food, and a smattering of heart-healthy items) is good to know about when Sunday brunch rolls around, especially if you have the kids in tow.

Clam Bar

$18

910 Bay Ave., Somers Point (609) 927-8783
at Annie Ave. at the Jersey Shore

Locally known as Smitty's, this low-atmosphere seafood joint is an old-timey "dive but no one cares," in light of its "beautiful setting" in the marina, "friendly and quick service," and simply "fantastic clam chowder." "Always crowded," it's "a great find" for "casual, good seafood," and what some call "the best cheap meal anywhere." BYOB, and dive in.

Clayton's

$39

65 E. Main St., Marlton (609) 985-5585
at Rt. 70 in So. Jersey

Victorian atmosphere abounds at this "quaint," "romantic" contemporary American with its soothing atmosphere, "perfect service," and glass-enclosed dining porch. "Elegant" yet casual dining includes veal dishes, rack of lamb, and Maryland crab, and while some of our reviewers note some "uneven performance in the kitchen," for most Clayton's is an all-around "enjoyable dining experience."

FOOD ROOM STAFF COST

Cotardo's

$26

1486 Blackwood-Clementon Rd., Cherrywood Plaza, Clementon (609) 627-2755 in So. Jersey

You get "a lot for your money" at this solid, down-to-earth Italian, located in Cherrywood Plaza on the Blackwood-Clementon pike. Known for pasta, seafood pescatore and coloring books for the kids, it's not a bad place when you want a quick, casual bite. BYOB.

Cousin's

$27

104 Asbury Ave., Ocean City (609) 399-9462
1st & Asbury at the Jersey Shore

"Save room for dessert"—and who could resist Killer Cake, peanut butter pie, or homemade eclairs?—at this locally popular Continental, serving a broad selection of "fab" veal, steak, seafood, pasta, and duck. Sunday breakfast and brunch and a bargain-priced twilight menu are added enticements at this comfortably casual restaurant, kin to the more famous Cousin's in Bargaintown.

Cousin's Country House

$37

Fire & Zion Rds., Egg Harbor Twp. (609) 927-5777
at the Jersey Shore

A lovely location near historic Bargaintown practically guarantees a following for this "elegant" European restaurant, set in a painstakingly renovated 150-year-old home complete with beamed ceilings, fireplaces, gazebo, and a waterfall. The extensive, eclectic menu never quite manages to catch up with the country-gentleman ambiance, but then again, how could it?

Crabby's

$23

1413 South Blvd. (Rt. 50), Belcoville (609) 625-2722
at Rt. 4050 in So. Jersey

Grab your mallets and dive into a pile of "the largest jumbo crabs ever" at this fun, ultra-"casual" crab house that specializes in all kinds of crabby creatures, from Maryland-style blue crabs to Dungeness and Alaskan king. Picnic tables and brown-paper place mats are about it for the decor, but all that is beside the point. There's all-you-can eat crabs for $17.95 on Wednesday, and a couple of other nightly fish fests, too. "Very enjoyable," "fun crowd."

Crab Pot

$26

9707 Amherst Ave , Margate (609) 823-1163
at Monroe St. at the Jersey Shore

"Sunset on the bay" and "great desserts" are just a few of the things that recommend this well-liked seafood restaurant that's right "on the water." Fans say it has "the best breakfast/brunch on the Shore," and they ought to know, since this "beautiful outdoor" spot gets pretty crowded in the morning (outdoor seating is strictly first-come-first-served, so arrive early to avoid disappointment). Steve's jumbo lump crab cakes and the "best lobster around" are specialties, but bring cash because Steve and Cookie don't take plastic.

Crab Trap

$27

2 Broadway, Somers Point (609) 927-7377
On the circle at the Jersey Shore

"Always crowded," this gigantic, Sixties-era Somers Point institution serves up "huge portions" of dependable seafood specialties amid a pleasantly fusty knotty-pine-nautical series of dining rooms. "Attentive" service, a friendly bar, and reasonable prices practically guarantee "a long line." It may not offer "the best seafood at the Shore," but the fact that it's open year-round is a decided plus at the shore.

Culinary Garden

$23

841 Central Ave., Ocean City (609) 399-3713
9th & Central at the Jersey Shore

No weekend in Ocean City would be complete without breakfast or brunch at this pretty, popular contemporary Continental-American located in a restored Victorian-era building in the heart of town. "They'll find a way to make you happy," with friendly service, delicious food, and charming ambiance. At dinner, you can BYOB to go along with traditional Shore favorites like crab cakes and chicken Maryland. Just watch out for seasonal hours.

David's Yellow Brick Toad

$34

1495 Hwy. 179, Lambertville (609) 397-3100, (800) The-Toad
in Central Jersey

"Good food" and "beautiful surroundings" make this older Continental-American a "great place for a leisurely dinner" or Sunday brunch to fortify you for a day of antiquing in Lambertville. "Awesome" views of gardens and surrounding farmlands provide the "best atmosphere," and there's a dining porch in season.

Deauville Inn

$23

201 Willard Rd., Strathmere (609) 263-2080
at Ocean Dr. at the Jersey Shore

"Great scenery" and dock-and-dine convenience on the bay between Ocean City and Sea Isle City set this otherwise-standard American-style eatery apart from other area joints. The moderately priced food may be merely "mediocre," but it's the "perfect place for late afternoon drinks," "crab night outside," or a "casual burger" on the deck. "You can go in anytime, all day," but insiders suggest you "bring your camera for the breathtaking sunsets."

Diamond's

$47

132 Kent St., Trenton (609) 393-1000
at Division St. in Central Jersey

Formality and high prices may attract an upscale clientele, but it does not necessarily make a great restaurant. The Italian and Continental food receives mixed reviews, with "just okay" the most appropriate comment in the bunch. Even more on the mark is "overpriced," for while they have 700 wines in the cellar and serve expensive aged beef, you're paying for it whether you order it or not.

FOOD ROOM STAFF COST

Dock's Oyster House

$32

2405 Atlantic Ave., Atlantic City (609) 345-0092
at Georgia Ave. at the Jersey Shore

In business since forever, A.C.'s oldest restaurant is this classic seafood standby offering funky pseudo-shipboard atmosphere (all teak walls and etched glass) and dependable fish and shellfish specialties. Though detractors grouse that there's "no ambiance," they're obviously the ones who prefer flash and glitter to old-line decor and friendly service. The piano bar attracts considerable crowds, too.

Doc's

$21

646 Bay Ave., Somers Point (609) 926-0404
across from Shore Memorial Hospital at the Jersey Shore

A "great find" in Somers Point, the primarily Continental menu of seafood, veal, chicken and pasta dishes pleases most diners, as does the relatively low price tag. Outdoor dining, overlooking the marina, allows for pipe and cigar smoking, and an attentive staff makes sitting on the deck at Doc's one of summer's simple pleasures.

Dutchman's Brauhaus

$23

2500 E. Bay Ave., Manahawkin (609) 494-6910
Manning Dr. in So. Jersey

LBI's only waterfront restaurant, this gemutlichkeit old-timer has a "great view" of Barnegat's lighthouse and its very own boat slips. Though a few suggest that the "quality of the food has gone down," if you "stick to the German specialties" and the dark weiss beer on tap you'll do fine. Reasonable prices, and an outdoor deck and raw bar are further enticements.

East Side Mario's

$17

1370 Blackwood-Clementon Rd., Clementon (609) 782-1969
in S. Jersey

This chain Italian takes atmosphere to movie set extremes—the whole place is done up like a Depression-era Little Italy streetside cafe, complete with old store fronts. Voters like the "boisterous, friendly" staff and "fun atmosphere," and say the food is "tasty and inexpensive." You can take kids, but the restaurant won't take reservations.

Ebbit Room

$47

25 Jackson St., Cape May (609) 884-5700
at the Jersey Shore

Quite possibly Cape May's "best dress-up restaurant," this drop-dead gorgeous contemporary American dining room in the lovingly restored Virginia Hotel wows its fans with innovative, well-executed food (the menu changes seasonally), sure-footed service, and a very nice wine list. Candlelight, cushy banquettes, and piano music add to the romantic atmosphere—and then you can slip away to your room right upstairs.

 = Superior = Excellent = Very Good

Farnsworth House

135 Farnsworth Ave., Bordentown (609) 291-9232
at Railroad Ave. in So. Jersey
"Quite a find" (if you can actually find it): "good food," a pretty setting in a 19th-century building in historic Bordentown, and "some of the nicest staff around." Of the creative, Italian/Mediterranean food, one fan enthuses, "every item tastes unique, and you can almost taste each individual item in it." Practically brand new, but certainly worth watching.

Ferry House

21 Ferry St., Lambertville (609) 397-9222
Union & Ferry in Central Jersey
Our participants say you'll find "world class" food at this Lambertville Contemporary American. With a more formal, candlelit dining room downstairs and an open bistro (piping in jazz and blues) upstairs, the Ferry House still only seats a little over fifty customers (soon to change with the addition of a patio). That, plus the "excellent" food and a cost-conscious BYO policy make reservations essential on the weekends.

Filomena

$24

1245 Blackwood-Clementon Rd., Commerce Plaza, Clementon (609) 784-6166 (at Kelly Dr. in So. Jersey)
Ignore the shopping-mall setting in favor of "excellent," reasonably priced Italian food served up family-style with roasted peppers, soup, and salad included in the price of all entrees. Family owned and operated, it serves up homemade pasta and nightly specials, and once you get inside the ambiance is pleasantly light and contemporary. One fan swears the "food is better than Philadelphia and half the price."

Flying W

$20

60 Forstertown Rd., Medford (609) 267-8787
at Rt. 541 in So. Jersey
Originally named for the dude-ranch-and-barn theme that dominated this 35-year-old restaurant & motel, they've managed to keep the name after a recent change to an aviation theme. Though its heyday may be over, this Medford giant is still "a great place to take the kids and watch the planes," especially during the all-you-can-eat buffets on Monday & Tuesday nights, and weekend brunch. The ultimate in kid friendly, you can even play shuffleboard.

Food For Thought

403 Haddon Ave., Haddonfield (609) 428-9839
at Kings Hwy. in So. Jersey
Tapestries and lace (and little rooms) and "excellent" Victorian decor help create a "terrific ambiance" at this teeny American in Haddonfield. The food is always "well-prepared," with grilled balsamic chicken and fish of the day being notable on the menu. The professional staff is happy to uncork the wine or beer you bring, but you have to call ahead to get a seat.

FOOD ROOM STAFF COST

Forsgate Country Club Dining Room

VOTE

Forsgate Dr., Jamesburg (908) 521-0070
NJ Tpk. exit 8-A in Central Jersey

Uppah, uppah class public dining room at the tiny Forsgate Country Club is where celebrants go for "beautifully presented" regional American cuisine, from a seasonal menu that features Black Angus beef and other primo treats. The views of the surrounding courses are splendid and the wine list gets a nod from the Wine Spectator, so why not make it a destination for the "wonderful" Sunday buffet brunch?

410 Bank Street

$38

410 Bank St., Cape May (609) 884-2127
at Lafayette St. at the Jersey Shore

One of the best restaurants on the Shore, and possibly in the state of New Jersey, is this quirky, thoroughly charming Louisiana/ Caribbean cafe, owned by Steve & Janet Miller and presided over by Asian chef Sing Cheng, who really knows his Creole. "Fabulous food" is matched only by the "fantastic" ambiance of this converted 1840s carriage house, with its atmospheric "outdoor dining area in summer" that might as well be in the French Quarter of New Orleans. BYOB, and watch out for seasonal hours.

Franco's Cafe

$26

7720 Ventnor Ave., Margate (609) 823-9019
at Douglas Ave. at the Jersey Shore

Linen and flowers elegantly punctuate this Italian spot in Margate, while a BYO policy and reasonable prices mark it as a good value. Seafood is the specialty of the house, and our voters say it is very fresh. "Great after the beach and a shower," they say, but warn that the no-reservation policy and crowding on weekends makes it necesssary to call ahead anyway.

Frenchtown Inn

$41

7 Bridge St., Frenchtown (908) 996-3300 (in Central Jersey)

One of the top restaurants in Central Jersey, chef/owner Robert Long's "romantic" nouvelle French "has it all," according to its legion of fans: "sophisticated" food, "attentive" staff and "elegant" yet "cozy" atmosphere. Sunday brunch is wonderful, and there's a more casual (and less expensive) Grill Room out back for when you're feeling less ambitious. No wonder so many of our Reporters are "always anxious to dine" at this "truly superb country inn." "Do make a trip"—but don't forget to reserve.

Frescos

$39

412 Bank St., Cape May (609) 884-0366
at Lafayette St. at the Jersey Shore

Newer sibling to next-door neighbor 410 Bank Street, this "romantic," BYOB regional Italian located in a restored Victorian home offers "outstanding" food only slightly "overshadowed" by "cramped" quarters and what could be a "long wait." Loyalists swear the Tuscan-style specialties like osso buco and homemade pasta are worth any inconvenience, however. The moral of the story: go early, go off-season, but go.

 = Superior = Excellent = Very Good

Friday's

$18

Princeton Market Fair Mall, Princeton (609) 520-0378 in Central Jersey
970 N. Rt. 73, Marlton (609) 596-9117 (in So. Jersey)
Rt. 40 & Tilton Rd., Pleasantville, NJ (609) 484-0999 in So. Jersey

Ignore the food rating and focus on the many honor spots this chain occupies in the front of our book. It is number 1 for bar food, number three for after-work drinks and children (we're guessing that one leads to the other) and is in the top ten for eavesdropping and even vegetarian menus. So what's the attraction? Most perceive it as a "run-of-the-mill singles restaurant," though admit the burgers and sandwiches are pretty good. Who knows? Someday this may be the only place to go for fried cheese.

Frog and the Peach

VOTE

29 Dennis St., New Brunswick (908) 846-3216 in Central Jersey

If you find yourself in New Brunswick, console yourself by visiting this "excellent," "very trendy" spot in a beautifully renovated old newspaper building. The decor is "new wave," the atmosphere is "bustling," and the "attentive" staff brings "excellent nouvelle" food in what everyone agrees is a "beautiful presentation." A cruvinet machine and lush appointments make the place a little pricey, but the no-children-after-6pm rule makes it a grown-up haven.

Full Moon

$22

23 Bridge St., Lambertville (609) 397-1096 Union St. in Central Jersey

Those who venture across the river from New Hope will find reasonable prices and innovative steak, seafood and pasta at this BYO spot in Lambertville. A good spot for Sunday brunch or dinner with the kids in tow.

Gary's Little Rock Cafe

$29

5212 Atlantic Ave., Ventnor (609) 823-2233 Atlantic & Little Rock at the Jersey Shore

New chef-owner Gary Pressman has made a "positive change" at this small, BYOB "gourmet American" that gets extra mentions for its "excellent warm duck salad" and caring staff. Though it's still a little too early to tell for sure, reports suggest that this could easily become a "great place at the beach."

Giumarello's

$29

512 Station Ave., Haddon Heights (609) 547-9393 at Rt. 30 (Whitehorse Pk.) in So. Jersey

A "favorite in South Jersey," this BYOB charmer in quaint Haddon Heights gets raves for its "consistently excellent" "gourmet Italian" food (especially the "great" bread), "good service," and "cheap early bird specials." Reservations may be "difficult," but once achieved you can expect a "delicious meal" at prices that reflect "the best value around."

FOOD ROOM STAFF COST

Greenbrier

$24

Rt. 70 & Haddonfield Rd., Cherry Hill (609) 662-0800
in So. Jersey

"Great weekend brunch" and a large selection of traditional and updated American favorites characterize this extremely popular spot in Cherry Hill. "Reasonable prices," "very good service," and lots of special features like a pre-theater (make that pre-race) and prix fixe dinners and a house credit card with frequent-diner privileges have made this comfortable area standby a local fixture for more than 40 years. Check out the great collection of local memorabilia—and come hungry for that six-course brunch.

Green Cuisine

$15

92nd St. & 3rd Ave., Stone Harbor (609) 368-1616
at the Jersey Shore

We thought that everyone on vacation always forgot their diet and splurged. Not so at this Stone Harbor health food spot, which serves natural foods, salads and sandwiches. Out-of-towners and locals alike "truly look forward" to the "very good," healthy food.

Gregory's

$20

900 Shore Rd., Somers Point (609) 927-6665
Delaware & Shore at the Jersey Shore

A circa-1908 dry-goods store and former house of ill repute (the rooms still have the beds and gaslamp fittings) is now home to a bustling, busy restaurant with a big, eclectic menu that runs the gamut from Mexican food and lobster dinners to bar food and one terrific hamburger. The 100-foot mahogany bar attracts a lively summertime crowd, but reasonable prices make Gregory's good for families too.

Hamilton's Grill Room

$37

8 Coryell St., Lambertville (609) 397-4343
bet. Lambert Ln. & Union St. in Central Jersey

For "Manhattan quality without the attitude," check out this "intimate," attractive little BYOB Mediterranean grill, specializing in hardwood-grilled fish and locally grown produce. "Super atmosphere," heads-up service, and a "creative" menu add up to an all-around "pleasant" experience. P.S. "the Boat House bar across the alley makes a great spot to go for an after-dinner drink."

Hardshell Cafe

$23

150 N. Rt. 73, Marlton (609) 983-3180
at Rt. 70 in So. Jersey

"Wonderful garlic crabs" and other fishy favorites make this exceedingly casual, inexpensive outpost of the Philadelphia original a South Jersey favorite when you feel like making a mess of things. Though some, er, crabby folks argue they'd "still go to Maryland," this one's a lot closer, and if "you bring the beer, they have the bucket."

 = Superior = Excellent = Very Good

Harvey Cedars Shellfish Co. $23

7904 Long Beach Blvd., Harvey Cedars (609) 494-7112
at the Jersey Shore

"True seashore dining in the rough" is yours at this inexpensive, seasonal seafood spot that's popular with locals and families. If you can't stand the crowds, there's a big takeout menu featuring the same "great food," but believe it or not, they don't serve dessert or coffee, whether you eat there or at home—and they don't serve liquor, either.

Hatteras Coastal Cuisine $31

801 Bay Ave., Somers Point (609) 926-3326
New Jersey & Bay Aves. at the Jersey Shore

"The gem of the Shore," this BYOB "Cape May-style charmer" makes a "wonderful addition" to an area that's long on restaurants but short on chef-owned contemporary American cafes. Crafted from an old Victorian house, chef-owner Bill Rollins' intensely personal restaurant features a "great menu" of seasonally changing fare, and his wife, Ellen, supervises a very well-trained staff. "A for effort and ambiance."

Henny's $27

9628 3rd Ave., Stone Harbor (609) 368-2929
at 96th St. at the Jersey Shore

This "excellent, everyday restaurant" is a "favorite summer hangout," with reliable-if-unexciting steak and seafood, "friendly" service, and fair prices. The decor is strictly nautical (read: trophy fish on the walls and loads of driftwood), but our Reporters like the clam chowder, the soft-shell crabs, and the casual, comfortable feel. A "joint," sure, but a "wonderful" one at that.

Houlihan's $18

Cherry Hill Mall, Cherry Hill (609) 662-9300 (in S. Jersey)

What to some is a great singles scene with great bar fare, is to others "chain food" in a "jazzed-up meat market." The concensus? "A good plastic place, slightly better than the competition."

Inn at Sugar Hill $37

5704 Mays Landing-Somers Point Rd., Mays Landing
(609) 625-2226 (Rts. 40 & 559 in So. Jersey)

Creative American food is the bill of fare at this Mays Landing dockside mini-inn. Overlooking the Great Egg Harbor River, this 150-year-old structure is better known for the ambiance and staff than for the food, but voters still call it "a favorite find in the pinelands." Though you can come by boat as well as by car, you still have to call ahead on weekends.

FOOD ROOM STAFF COST

Italian Bistro

$22

Ocean One Mall, Atlantic City (609) 345-8799
at the Jersey Shore

"Surprisingly good," writes one voter. Well, creativity would be a surprise from an Italian Bistro with this name. "A great place for all," meaning families, say reviewers, though they are more inclined to talk about this mini-chain's more exotic locations, like "in the Ocean Mall in Atlantic City." The "nice bar" has an above-average selection of wines by the glass, and the pastries are also recommended. No reservations taken.

Jackson Mountain Cafe

$21

400 Washington St., Cape May (609) 884-5648
Jackson St. & Washington St. Mall at the Jersey Shore

It's about people-watching and "casual, relaxed" atmosphere at this otherwise underwhelming family-friendly cafe-bar with a prime sidewalk location on the Washington Street Mall, Cape May's lively shopping promenade. Gourmets say "stay away," but it's actually "great for lunch," especially when you have too little time and too many kids. Lower your expectations and order a burger.

J.B. Winberie

$19

1 Palmer Square, Princeton (609) 921-0700 (in Central Jersey)

These chain Americans are popular with students, because the food is "inexpensive," the atmosphere is "relaxed," the servers are "friendly," and some locations have outdoor dining. The ratings are low, but you know what to expect: "stick to burgers and salads."

Joe Italiano's

$24

6126 Black Horse Pk., Mays Landing (609) 625-1181 (in So. Jersey)

"Joe's ambiance is nothing special" report our reviewers, "but the pasta is superb!" This Mays Landing Italian has fans from all over, who come for the "consistent quality food," and the little touches. Everything is cooked to order, and even the takeout is specially wrapped and includes salad and garlic bread. You'll want to take out, unless you don't mind the tight quarters.

Joe's Peking Duck House

$18

145 Rt. 73 S. (Behind Olga's Diner), Marlton (609) 985-1551
at Rt. 70 E. in So. Jersey

"No atmosphere," no credit cards, no liquor license—but "excellent" Cantonese food, including Hong Kong-style dim sum, "speedy service," and low prices keep Joe's "busy," "noisy," and "good." Needless to say, the eponymous Peking duck has garnered considerable local notice. P.S. Vegetarians will be particularly happy here.

Jo Jo's Pizzeria

$18

6501 Ventnor Ave., Ventnor (609) 822-6475
at Newport Ave. at the Jersey Shore

Family-friendly and very inexpensive, this low-key BYOB Southern Italian has been owned by the Cannuscio clan for three generations—with the loyal local following to prove it. It's not much to look at, but the family-style portions are huge, and the restaurant stays open until the relatively late hour of 11. The booming takeout business is another plus.

Kamakura

$27

270 N. Elmwood Rd., Marlton (609) 983-2990
at Rt. 70 in So. Jersey

When in Marlton, do as the Japanese do at this authentic, if modern Japanese restaurant, that consistently wins the praise of our voters and awards from local and state-wide publications. You will have a "transforming experience into another culture," with very high marks all around, and atmosphere that includes a Tatami room and Japanese gardens. For a warm night of show tunes, they also have a fireplace and Karaoke at the bar.

Katie O'Brien's

$23

427 Crystal Lake Ave., Haddon Twp. 609-858-2253
McCarthy Blvd. in So. Jersey

Fun is the M.O. of this American eclectic, known more as an Irish bar than a real restaurant. Those few who know it note the "beautiful" pub and "landscaped outdoor dining," but for the record there's also darts, Saturday-night entertainment, and a menu that runs the gamut from burgers to fajitas.

Knife & Fork Inn

$37

Atlantic & Pacific Aves., Atlantic City (609) 344-1133
at the Jersey Shore

"Atlantic City squared" resides at this sentimental "favorite" that pleases fans despite—or perhaps because of—"snooty owners," staid surroundings, and an "expensive," all-American seafood menu. It "never changed" for 68 years, but we get the feeling its largely-older clientele doesn't mind a bit. Why should they, with dependable food, hardworking staff, and more old-line shore atmosphere than you can shake a stick at?

La Campagne

$41

312 Kresson Rd., Cherry Hill (609) 429-7647
Brace & Marlcress Rds. in So. Jersey

"Wonderful" farmhouse atmosphere and "exciting," "creative" country French food distinguish this romantic little Cherry Hill restaurant, which has a lovely outdoor patio when the weather's fine. Inside, candles and firelight glow on antiques and polished floors, and the staff is sure-footed and kind. Desserts and tasting menus are special pleasures, and BYOB helps keep otherwise-highish prices in line. Small wonder it's one of our Reporters' Top 5 Favorites in Jersey.

= Good **= Fair** **[no rating] = Poor**

FOOD ROOM STAFF COST

La Familia Sonsini

$28

202 Old Marlton Pk., Medford (609) 654-5217 (Hartford Rd. in So. Jersey)
Step back in time to this well-rated little Sonsini-family-owned BYOB cafe that reflects its owners' roots in Italy and Louisiana. The comfortable, old-world atmosphere reflects kindly on the Creole-Italian menu specialities, and the service is friendly and attentive.

Lahiere's

VOTE

11 Witherspoon St., Princeton (609) 921-2798
Off Nassau St. in Central Jersey
Voters like the "tweedy atmosphere" at this upscale American restaurant. After all, it's located in Princeton. The food scores solid marks, but the price is high, presumably due in part to the large, award-winning wine list. While reviewers say it is comfortable, don't forget to wear a jacket at dinner, it's required, as are reservations.

Lambertville Station

$30

11 Bridge St., Lambertville (609) 397-8300 (in Central Jersey)
"Great atmosphere" in a restored Victorian-era train station and an "interesting, different menu" (heavy on the unusual game in season) make this a "must-see" in the touristy New Hope-Lambertville area. Early bird specials and the brunch buffet are a "great deal," and if the decor is a little Disney-esque, our reviewers don't seem to mind a bit. Best tip: "fun during shad festival."

Le Palais

$46

1133 Boardwalk, Merv Griffin's Resorts, Atlantic City
(609) 340-6400 (at the Jersey Shore)
"Make sure you have your requests ready for the singer" at this "supper club of royal standards" located in Merv Griffin's Resorts. The "lovely, elegant" French food is hardly a match for the swanky red-velvet-and-chandelier ambience and, oh, yes, did we mention the entertainment? Pricey and somewhat "pompous," Le Palais is nonetheless one of the better dress-up options in A.C.

Library II

$34

306 Rt. 73, Voorhees (609) 424-0198 (in So. Jersey)
"The best salad bar" and "great steaks" make this 10-year-old institution "heaven" for a no-big-deal night out. It's very busy, but "worth the wait if you're in the mood" for high-quality steak that's cut to order and priced by the ounce. (There's also prime rib, king crab, and surf-and-turf.) And did we mention that "unbeatable" salad bar?

Library III

$27

6605 Black Horse Pk., Cardiff (609) 645-7655 (in So. Jersey)
Part of the immensely popular (and independently owned) Library system, this "fantastic" steakhouse's shtick is good-quality meat that you order directly from the chef and pay for by the ounce, plus a huge salad bar to forage through while you wait. The open kitchen and library decor add to the dining-event-as-spectator-sport feel. Not an intellectual experience, certainly, but not bad when you're in the right mood.

 = Superior = Excellent = Very Good

Little Saigon

$16

2801 Arctic Ave., Atlantic City (609) 347-3577
Arctic & Iowa at the Jersey Shore

"Go for the excellent food" at this tiny, low-atmosphere Vietnamese "gem" located in a fringey A.C. neighborhood. "Very good hosts and staff," under the supervision of chef-owner Lien Pham make Little Saigon "a happy place," specializing in authentic dishes like shrimp hot pot, beef wrapped in grape leaves, and stir-fried chicken with lemon grass. No plastic and no liquor, but at these prices who's complaining?

Lobster House

$33

Fisherman's Wharf, Cape May (609) 884-8296
at Rt. 109 at the Jersey Shore

"Unmistakably Shore"—"long waits," lobster dinners, "wonderful views of the harbor" and all. Dock and dine on the boat deck, grab a table in the huge informal dining room, or avoid the crowds with takeout from the retail store. Whether you find the decor tacky or atmospheric, and the food from the giant menu "delicious" or "overrated," is a matter of some debate, but after 60 years in business, they must be doing something right.

Lobster Loft

$28

42nd & Bay, Sea Isle City (609) 263-3000
at the Jersey Shore

Vacationers say "the fish is best at Lobster Loft" in Sea Isle City, overlooking the inland waterway, where you can eat indoors or outdoors. This seasonal restaurant specializes, naturally, in the king of crustaceans (try the lobster fra diavolo), and don't be afraid to bring the kids—there's plenty to keep them occupied while you choose your lobster from the dining room tank.

Lone Star Steakhouse & Saloon

$28

1521 Blackhorse Pk., Turnersville (609) 262-1737
in So. Jersey

Part of a nationwide chain of insanely popular, Texas-themed steakeries, this "place for beef" attracts hordes with its reasonable prices (for steak anyway) and fun, family-friendly country-and-western ambiance. Ruth's Chris it ain't, but if this one doesn't "put you in the mood for great beef and beer," better check your pulse. Heed this warning: No reservations are taken, so be prepared to wait.

Longport Inn

$29

3103 Atlantic Ave , Longport 609-822-5435
31st Ave. at the Jersey Shore

New owners are intent on making over this venerable Longport American, whittling down the long but lackluster menu and adding French and Continental fine-dining touches. Though voters are comfortable with the tavern atmosphere in the bar, there's plenty of room for improvement on the food scores.

FOOD ROOM STAFF COST

Loose Ends

$29

517 Station Ave., Haddon Heights (609) 546-9777
at the White Horse Pk. in So. Jersey

"A little innovative," a little "different," this small, intensely personal little BYO cafe specializes in chef Annemarie Bertino's creative, internationally influenced cooking. Caring service and fresh, homemade food, including delicious desserts, make this "always one of the best" for the type of diner who is more concerned with a good meal than a dining experience.

Lorenzo's

VOTE

66 S. Clinton Ave., Trenton (609) 695-6868
Across from RR station in Central Jersey

Right across from the train station in Trenton, Pete Lorenzo's has been serving Steaks and Italian specialties to an upscale crowd of families, politicos, businessmen, and "family" for as long as our voters can remember. The old charm of the place is reflected in the dark bar, the "big martinis" and other stiff drinks, the expertly-aged beef and the classic (if heavy) menu items. Be warned: it is popular and noisy, and if you get stuck in the newer rooms, you might feel like you're in a suburban rec room.

Los Amigos

$20

1926 Atlantic Ave., Atlantic City (609) 344-2293
bet. Michigan & Ohio at the Jersey Shore

This Atlantic City Mexican, already popular for its all-day happy-hour drink prices and "the best margaritas in Atlantic City," has added a new menu that's "more Tex-Mex style—great value with some unique items." The room doesn't take any prizes, but it doesn't seem to deter the wee-hours casino crowd.

Louisa's

$26

104 Jackson St., Cape May (609) 884-5882
at Washington St. at the Jersey Shore

Our reporters are loath to rave about this wonderful little chef-owned cafe that's been around since before Cape May became a dining Mecca: "It's getting more and more difficult to get a table!" The "limited menu" of eclectic, internationally influenced food is always good for the "highest rating," but "crowded seating" and "standing in line" is almost guaranteed at a place that has only 20 seats. Totally charming, but if you don't like waiting, don't come in August. Bring your own wine, a good sense of humor—and cash.

Mad Batter

$28

19 Jackson St., Carroll Villa Hotel, Cape May (609) 884-5970
Beach & Lafayette at the Jersey Shore

"Ask for a front-porch table" and settle in for some "great people-watching" at this lively, eclectic little BYOB spot that's practically "de rigeuer for brunch in Cape May." Though a few people say the "description of the food is better than the taste," for most the "creative" menu and "lovely" setting in the Victorian-era Carroll Villa Hotel make this a "best spot on the Shore."

 = Superior = Excellent = Very Good

Malaga

$25

511 Lalor St., Hamilton Twp. (609) 396-8878
at Hewitt St. in Central Jersey

While Philadelphians may lament the need for more good Spanish restaurants, South Jerseyans are laughing all the way to Hamilton Township, for "large portions" of "excellent Spanish food" from occasional tapas to their standby, seafood paella. Lowfat menu options have some reviewers questioning the authenticity of the food, but this is the '90s, even in Spain.

Mama Ventura's

$36

178 Rt. 73, Voorhees (609) 767-7400
in So. Jersey

Thirty-two years old and counting, what some call the "best Italian in South Jersey" still has a loyal, family-intensive following for old-line veal, chicken, seafood, and pasta dishes. Nineties touches include Wednesday Ladies' Night and a band on weekends, and Thursday is Italian night, complete with a tacky-but-fun sing along.

Mansion on Main Street

$31

Main St., Plaza 3000, Voorhees (609) 751-6060
in So. Jersey

The "elegant Sunday brunch buffet extravaganza" is what our reviewers remember first about this otherwise "mediocre" Continental. It's not a mansion at all, but an overblown catering-hall-cum-corporate retreat located at the back of a mixed-use development in suburban Voorhees (the only other time it's open to the public is for the Wednesday-night international buffet). There's a gazebo, swan pond and waterfalls for photo ops, of course. Not bad if you like a big breakfast; otherwise, forget it.

Marriott's Seaview Resort

$38

401 S. New York Rd., Absecon (609) 652-1800
Jimmy Leeds Rd. & Rt. 9 at the Jersey Shore

Known for its "spectacular Friday-night seafood spread"—$37.50, and what a way to go!—this classy Continental dining room in an upscale resort is a good bet when you want to get far from A.C.'s madding crowds. (The champagne brunch buffet is a downright steal for $21.95). White-glove service and elegant atmosphere that includes a rotunda ceiling and huge chandeliers keeps the riff-raff out. There's also a more casual steak-and-brew pub if you want to mingle.

Mastoris Diner

$19

144 Rt. 130, Bordentown (609) 298-4650
in So. Jersey

"Number one in the Diner Hall of Fame" is this big-menu Bordentown tradition, "worth the trip" or a "turnpike detour" for "generous portions" (some say "grossly large") of straight-up American food at "bargain prices." Desserts, homemade cinnamon buns, and "breads to die for" claim special merit, and it's open until 1 A.M. (2 A.M. on weekends) if you get the post-midnight munchies.

Maureen

$41

Beach & Decatur Sts., Cape May (609) 884-3774 (Jersey Shore)

Owners "Steve and Maureen Horn turn an evening into art" at this lovely seashore dining spot that started the culinary renaissance in Cape May. The Victorian atmosphere is a draw, especially on the Atlantic-view porch, and Steve Horn's internationally influenced contemporary American food (though expensive) can be "extraordinary." An interesting wine list and heads-up service also recommend it.

Medici at the Sands

VOTE

Indiana Ave. & Brighton Park, A.C. (609) 441-4200 at the Shore

One of the luxest places on the Boardwalk, this dressy, European-style Italian does a commendable job with specialties like veal Milanese and balsamic-grilled lamb chops. It's not cheap, no, but for sophisticated dining after a big win, you could do worse.

Meil's

$26

Bridge & Main Sts., Stockton (609) 397-8033 (in Central Jersey)

Nobody seems to mind the "close quarters" at this Regional American restaurant in Stockton, and even say it's "worth the wait." It's perfect for weekend lunch while visiting Bucks County nearby, because the "creative," "down-home cooking" is "plentiful and fun." With an on-site bakery and lots of great comfort food, "eat until it aches you."

Melissa's Bistro

$29

9307 Ventnor Ave., Margate (609) 823-1414
1 block from Lucy the Elephant at the Jersey Shore

A sweet little French-style bistro (antiques, lace curtains, flowers on every table) is the setting for chef-owner Melissa Lavin's eclectic, New Age menu, which highlights organic produce, home-grown herbs, and delicious desserts. Bring your own wine to complement Melissa's lovely, light-touch food.

Mexican Food Factory

$21

601 W. Rt. 70, Marlton (609) 983-9222 (in So. Jersey)

"Best Mexican food in South Jersey" may be faint praise indeed for this loud, gaudy margarita mill that packs 'em in for traditional tacos, burritos, and enchiladas, plus a few "Southwestern fusion" dishes like smoked turkey quesadillas and ancho-crusted tuna, but the Mexican Food Factory gets an awful lot of votes from our reviewers. Patio dining, South-of-the-border guitar music, and a kid-friendly atmosphere don't hurt any.

Mrs. London's Cafe

$32

515 Rt. 73 S., Meadows Edge Marketplace, Marlton
(609) 983-7744 (in So. Jersey)

"A wonderful evening" is yours at this "lovely" little chef-owned cafe located in soothing, Victorian-style quarters in Marlton. The well-rated, internationally accented food is judged "always good," and it's matched by gracious service and a comfortable, homey atmosphere. In short, "everything about Mrs. London's" is a pleasure.

Nonna's

VOTE

Haddonfield-Berlin Rd., Cherry Hill (609) 795-1778
Brace Rd. in So. Jersey

This new Tuscan opened too late for many Romac Reporters to draw a bead on it. The few who did found "excellent steak" and "good ambiance." The ceilings are high, and there's a bright, airy room to the side that looks perfect for private parties.

Obadiah's

$33

321 Roosevelt Blvd., Marmora (609) 390-3574
On causeway to Ocean City at the Jersey Shore

This is the upscale side, connected to the crabhouse called O.B.'s, where you can get a drink or sit if you arrived dressed too casually for Obadiah's. It's a little more upscale than most other shore restaurants, with a professional staff, but like many other seasonal spots, it's only open from May to September.

Old Swedes Inn

VOTE

301 Kings Highway, Swedesboro (609) 467-2052 (Rt. 322 in S. Jersey)

Our voters tell us they find "very good food" at this New American and French Provincial restaurant in Swedesboro. "Quiet and romantic," with classical and light music in the background, it's a "super" atmosphere that's also kid-friendly, with 1/2 portions on the grill menu for the little ones. P.S. The staff is called "special."

Olga's Diner

$15

Rts. 70 & 73, Marlton (609) 596-1700 (in So. Jersey)

What constitutes "the best diner selection" does not necessarily a great restaurant make: so what? Our voters tell us they've "never had a bad meal," and like the great diners of the ages, it has "great late night grub and atmosphere." Olga's is a landmark, if not for the "diversified salad bar items," then for the fact that it's halfway to the shore.

Outback Steakhouse

$24

230 E. Lake Dr., Cherry Hill (609) 482-1350 (in S. Jersey)

This Steak chain is clearly popular—why else would so many voters complain so bitterly about long waits (up to two hours at times) for a table? Many feel the steaks are "good for a chain" and rave about the whole, batter-dipped "bloomin' onion." Others say it is just "Rustler with an accent" and "way overrated." The restaurant's dinner-only hours make it "not very user-friendly." The concensus? "Good steak fun" after a "cows to slaughter" wait.

Owl Tree

$29

2323 New Rd., Northfield (609) 645-0066 (at the Jersey Shore)

Something for everyone is the name of the game at this A.C.-area fern bar, from burgers and prime rib to Italian and Mexican specialties. Sister to the original Owl Tree in Harvey Cedars, the mainland version also sports fair prices and a lively-but-older bar scene.

= Good **= Fair** **[no rating] = Poor**

FOOD ROOM STAFF COST

Oyster Creek Inn

$20

41 N. Oyster Creek Rd., Leed's Point (609) 652-8565
at Rt. 9 at the Jersey Shore

"A hidden treasure" in Leed's Point, says one voter about this large, family-owned American, with a great view of the nearby wildlife refuge, but from what we hear about the room, you'll want to spend your time looking out the windows anyway. Believe it or not, a nautical theme, with fishnets and seafaring pictures on the walls, sometimes doesn't work.

Pasta Blitz by Lamberti

$20

1888 Rt. 70 E., Cherry Hill (609) 424-4817
at Springdale Rd. in So. Jersey

With tighter quarters than its Philadelphia cousins across the river, folks find this member of the Lamberti family unable to live up to the usually reliable name. Still, it's cheaper than most, due to the many nightly specials and a BYO policy, and you don't have to feel uncomfortable about taking the kids.

Peaches at Sunset

$32

1 Sunset Blvd., West Cape May (609) 898-0100
Sunset Blvd. & Broadway at the Jersey Shore

Romac Rule #1136: Restaurants with gift shops just don't have good food. Romac Rule #1137: Rules were meant to be broken. Everyone who has visited this Cape May Continental and Eclectic restaurant agrees that the "great funky food" is "very good." Add to that all the bells and whistles of frequent diner cards and early bird buy-one, get-one-free specials, and you've got a loyal following of diners, proudly sporting "Peaches" sun visors.

Peter Shield's

$38

1301 Beach Dr., Cape May (609) 884-6491
at Trenton Ave. at the Jersey Shore

With a view of the beach, and the Atlantic Ocean beyond, this Cape May French American attracts an upscale crowd for special meals on holidays, or any other time of the year. We hear there's a provincial feel, with a fireplace, copper kettles, and a lovely porch for summer dining. Dress up, and don't forget to call ahead for reservations, especially on weekends. Those who have been there say they "must go back."

Pirates Inn

$28

Centerton Rd., Mt. Laurel (609) 235-5737, (800) 70-PIRATE
Exit 43 off Rt. 295 in So. Jersey

Theme-park central is the name of the game at this big waterfront steak-and-fish place located on the Rancocas River, complete with pirate ships docked outside. Too bad the food ranges from fair to "awful," because the nautical atmosphere might appeal to the kiddies. The bottom line, as one review puts it, might be: "great for lunch, lousy for dinner."

Planet Hollywood

$24

2100 Pacific Ave., Caesar's Atlantic City, Atlantic City (609) 347-7827 (Arkansas & The Boardwalk at the Jersey Shore)

If you haven't heard of this big, memorabilia-packed California/American chain, we hope you're enjoying that rock you're living under. The movie-and television-inspired "atmosphere is just wonderful," packed with "fun celebrity paraphernalia," particularly from the films of shareholders Sly, Arnold, Demi and Bruce. Be warned, "the wait is forever," but "worth it," especially for the Cap'n Crunch chicken fingers.

Point Pub

$24

Rt. 9 & Bethel Rd., Somers Point Shopping Plaza, Somers Point (609) 927-2491 (at the Jersey Shore)

Named for the Town of Somers Point, this restaurant has been serving steaks, pasta and seafood for more than ten years, though our voters don't think it is anything special. You could give it a shot if you're in town, but with these ratings, what's the point?

Ponzio's Kingsway

$18

7 W. Rt. 70, Cherry Hill (609) 428-4808 at Rt. 41 in So. Jersey

"The place to stop for breakfast" on the way to LBI, this "consistently good" diner-cum-restaurant on the King's Highway circle has been attracting hordes for 30 years. "Great" coffee, "memorable" French toast, and "good," "fresh" American food at prices that are "not expensive," to say the least, are what keeps Ponzio's popular. Friendly service doesn't hurt, either.

Pub, The

$24

Airport Circle, Pennsauken (609) 665-6440 Rts. 130, 38, 70 in So. Jersey

Around since the fifties (and it looks it), The Pub is "still the big steakhouse" in the area, with a "superb" salad bar, "the best baked potatoes," "great steaks" from the "open hearth," and prices that represent a "good deal for the money." It appeals to an older clientele, of course, who claim you can "recapture your youth" at this paean to "another tradition gone with the wind." "Affordable" and "comfortable," and that's the bottom line.

Ram's Head Inn

$40

9 W. White Horse Pk., Absecon (609) 652-1700 U.S. Rt. 30 & Garden State Pkwy. at the Jersey Shore

"Very good fine dining" can be had at this "lovely," "very expensive" Colonial-style classic Continental, owned by the Knowles family since 1978. It can be "wedding city," yes, but the numbers indicate that for most of our reviewers, this is "an outstanding restaurant," with "elegant" service, well-rated food (local produce and game a specialty) and views of the formal gardens and a pretty courtyard. Gentlemen, you can leave your tie behind, but don't forget your jacket.

FOOD ROOM STAFF COST

Red, Hot & Blue

$19

Rt. 70 & Sayer Ave., Cherry Hill (609) 665-7427 (in So. Jersey)
"If you love ribs and blues," says one Romac Reporter of this Memphis-style barbecue spot in Cherry Hill, then "this is the place." With live music Thursdays through Saturdays, and kids-eat-free and other early bird specials, "the clientele gets into the bands and everyone is extremely friendly!"

Remi's Cafe

$21

141 Kings Hwy. E., Haddonfield (609) 795-7232 at Haddon Ave. in So. Jersey
This Italian on Haddonfield's historic Main Street offers casual but romantic dining on classic Italian dishes (veal saltimbucca is a specialty) in a candlelit room. The ratings aren't eye-opening, but the reasonable prices are.

Renault A'top the Winery

$39

72 N. Bremen Ave., Egg Harbor City (609) 965-2111 (in So. Jersey)
"You can always expect quality" from this "romantic" creative American manse, located in the Renault Winery and surrounded by vineyards and woods. The pricey food is dubbed "excellent," and so is the service and the setting. Stained glass windows, wine-barrel booths, and rooms full of antiques add to the atmosphere. Sunday brunch is a best bet, attracting supplicants from far and wide.

Richard's Natural Foods

VOTE

10 White Horse Rd., Voorhees (609) 627-5057 at Burnt Mill Rd. in So. Jersey
The mostly Thirtysomething crowd that goes to this macrobiotic Vegetarian (including fish) has great things to say about the healthy cooking. "You feel energized by the well-prepared, healthy food," going as far as to say it's "the best vegetarian there is." There are even classes available, and the lectures, combined with the new age music, might account for the low response to the ambiance.

Sack O Subs

$10

5217 Ventnor Ave, Ventnor (609) 823-2552 at Little Rock at the Shore
Voters find the "best Italian sub" (don't call them hoagies here) and "best cheesesteak in the world" at this Ventnor sandwich shop, which will even fix up a grilled vegetable sandwich for vegetarians.

Sagami

$27

Rt. 130, Collingswood (609) 854-9773 (in So. Jersey)
Tops in New Jersey, whether the criteria is Japanese or not, Sagami is "one of the best sushi spots nationwide" according to the many Reporters who commented on this "wonderful place, warm, friendly, and tasty." "Fresh sushi and sashimi" is the hallmark, of course, but the rest of the menu is good, too, ensuring a large, devoted clientele. The "great Japanese atmosphere" is enhanced by fair prices, and the "best use of beautiful ceramic dishes, bowls, etc." around. P.S. It's BYOB, and you can "bring your own sake, which they'll heat up for you."

Sage Diner $17

1170 Rt. 73, Mt. Laurel (609) 727-0770
at Church Rd. in So. Jersey

You get "lots of food" at this Continental Seafooder in Mt. Laurel, and while it's "not bad," the quality is actually better than you find at most places that serve breakfast anytime. The big story is the "reasonable tab," low enough to bring the whole family, but you'll have to pretend to make it feel like a special occasion. Sage diners bring their own wine or beer.

Sailfish Cafe (Glenning's Sailfish Cafe) $20

7805 Ventnor Ave., Margate (609) 822-6311
at Essex at the Jersey Shore

"One-of-a-kind" describes this ultra-casual spot, with its inexpensive, trendy menu, TV-intensive sports bar, and off-and-on schedule of dancing, trivia, and Karaoke. Food and service will never win any prizes, but the kid-friendly dining and late-night bar hours really hit the spot in beachy Margate.

Samuel's $27

178 S. White Horse Pk., Berlin (609) 753-0544
at Taunton Rd. in So. Jersey

"Samuel's food is out of this world," say those who know of this "surprisingly good" international-style restaurant located in a historic Victorian setting. Sure-footed service and a nice prix fixe dinner are added attractions, but the real winner is the delicious Sunday brunch. BYOB helps keep the tab reasonable.

Scannicchio's $30

119 S. California Ave., Atlantic City (609) 348-6378
at Pacific Ave. at the Jersey Shore

This Italian American in Atlantic City seems like the kind of place you'll fall in love with (because love is blind), or you'll move on in search of greener pastures. The radio supplies most of the atmosphere, and reports on the kitchen are mixed. Our voters say the staff could try harder, a surprise to us from what we've seen in recent press.

Screnci's $24

6208 Landis Ave., Sea Isle City (609) 263-2217
63rd. & Landis at the Jersey Shore

This Italian American Seafooder in Sea Isle City may not stand head and shoulders above the many other good ones at the shore, but they do go the extra mile to deliver the standard dishes at a bargain, if you know what to look for. "Byob appeals" to the moneywise, as do the early bird and prix fixe specials. Call ahead for an evening of garlic, parmesan, and Frankie on the stereo.

FOOD ROOM STAFF COST

Sea Grill

$33

225 21st St., Avalon (609) 967-5511
at Dune Dr. at the Jersey Shore

This Avalon Steak and Seafooder is a blend of fish market, butcher, and haute cuisine. You wait in line and order your meal through a window to the kitchen. If you want steak, you pay by the ounce. Then you grab a plate and hit the salad bar, again serving yourself. You can order from a choice of 15 wines by the glass to enjoy along with your "very good," expertly prepared meal. Of course the "service is quick" at this "noisy" place—what else does the staff have to do?

Siri's Thai French

$25

2117-2119 Rt. 70 W., Cherry Hill (609) 663-6781
Across from the Garden State Park in So. Jersey

While it may be "on a drab strip on Route 70" (across from the Garden State Park), that doesn't take away from the "sophisticated, elegant interior." Called "a smash from the night it opened," they have the "best Thai food there is," at least in Cherry Hill. "Packed on weekends," voters appreciate the "good ambiance and prices," the BYO policy, and put this place in the top 40 on our poll for food.

Som Sak Thai Cuisine

$19

200 Whitehorse Rd., Echo Shoppes, Voorhees (609) 782-1771
at Rt. 30 in So. Jersey

If you haven't had Som Sak lately, one voter recommends you try it again, they "show steady improvement." It would be tough for them to get much higher marks for their "very good" Thai dishes, with creative specialties like Crispy Red Snapper. Served by an "excellent" and professional staff, they also have many vegetarian specials. It's fairly inexpensive, with a byo policy, and lunch is a real bargain.

Stockton Inn

$41

1 Main St., Stockton (609) 397-1250 (Bridge St. in Central Jersey)

"Wonderful, cozy, and romantic," this historic Stockton Continental inspired Rogers & Hart to write the song "There's a small hotel with a wishing well." A trout pond, five fireplaces, a garden bar, and an "unbelievable outdoor setting with a waterfall" add to the lovingly restored 18th century atmosphere, and the staff "knows how to please customers." "For a real romantic treat," our Reporters "would recommend" it, especially for Sunday brunch in the gardens. All this and lodging, too, make the Stockton Inn a "favorite."

Sweetwater Casino

$28

2780 7th Ave., Sweetwater (609) 965-3285
7th Ave. & Rt. 623 in So. Jersey

"What a view" of the marina and the Mullica River at this comfortable, old-line seafood and steak specialist (crab Imperial, fried oysters and chicken salad—you know the drill) that's been in business since the 1920s. You can dance in your Docksiders or dine outside on the deck. The food can be "disappointing," but considering the dearth of competition and the abundance of old-fashioned atmosphere, what's the point of complaining?

 = Superior **= Excellent** **= Very Good**

Tabernacle Inn $24

1488 Rt. 206, Tabernacle (609) 268-1060
Medford Lakes Rd. & Rt. 532 in So. Jersey
While the post-and-beam construction (made with wood from Utah, no less) creates a Cathedral-like atmosphere in this holy spot next to the Wharton State Forest in Tabernacle, the Eclectic food, focusing mainly on French, Italian and modern American dishes, is a less-than-religious experience for most. Dress up, and try the champagne buffet at Sunday brunch after church.

Tony's Baltimore Grill $15

2800 Atlantic Ave., Atlantic City (609) 345-5766
at Iowa Ave. at the Jersey Shore
"Do not underestimate this legendary Shore family restaurant" say in-the-know reviewers who laud its "relaxed" atmosphere, "good, plain Italian food" ("great pizza") and down-to-earth service. Yeah, it's not much to look at and they take no plastic, but considering that it may be the "cheapest, tastiest secret of A.C.," who's complaining?

Tortilla Flats $21

2540 Dune Dr., Avalon (609) 967-5658
at 25th St. at the Jersey Shore
Chef-owner Jeffrey Schwartz' menu at this Avalon Southwestern goes beyond basics to dishes like blue tortilla crab cakes and grilled chicken with black bean sauce, prompting some Romac Reporters to call it "the best Mexican down the shore." Open President's Day weekend to Thanksgiving weekend.

Tre Figlio $34

500 W. Whitehorse Pk., Egg Harbor City (609) 965-3303
at Manheim Ave. in So. Jersey
Who would have guessed that you could find a "culinary gem" in this odd spot on the White Horse Pike? The "sophisticated" Italian food, family-friendly service, and casually elegant atmosphere (check out the Bacchus murals on the walls) make it "well worth leaving the shore" when you're in the mood for homemade pasta (lobster ravioli is a specialty of the house), fresh seafood, and one "world-class double-cut veal chop." Ciao, bella.

Tulipano Nero $27

3747 Church Rd., Rite Aid Shopping Ctr., Mt. Laurel
(609) 235-6955
at Fellowship Rd. in So. Jersey
"Excellent and reliable food" and "courteous service" are the reason this elegantly casual Northern Italian wins high marks in all categories from our reporters. The open grill and wood-burning oven in the center of the dining room set the stage for a very "nice" evening indeed, and there's "good value when you bring your own wine." One know-it-all says you can "come here to see the Mob," but you didn't hear it from us.

FOOD ROOM STAFF COST

Ugly Mug $17

426 Washington Street Mall, Cape May (609) 884-3459
at the Jersey Shore

"The place to hang out in Cape May all day long—especially when it's raining," this cheap, cash-only burger-joint-cum-bar takes its name from the hundreds and hundreds of customer-donated mugs that festoon the ceiling (if you own a mug, you can drink "great beer" out of it for just 50 cents). The food is exceedingly straightforward, but it's a "fun place to people-watch," especially during tacky-to-the-max events like the U.S. National Froth Blowing Championship. Best U.M. trivia: if the mug faces the ocean, its owner is deceased.

Urie's Fish Fry $32

588 Old Rio Grande Ave., Wildwood (609) 522-4947
Rio Grande at the foot of Bridge at the Jersey Shore

Located on the intracoastal waterway which goes all the way to Florida, this huge, hoppin' '50s-era "madhouse with food" packs them in for dependable-if-unsurprising all-American seafood, dished out in huge quantities for events like the Hawaiian Luau (watch out for the Polynesian Revue). There's an outdoor canopied deck in season, and just in case you care, a gift shop with a "wide variety of items for every gift occasion."

Urie's Reef & Beef $29

488 W. Rio Grande Ave., Wildwood (609) 522-7761
Rio Grande & Susquehanna at the Jersey Shore

Not to be confused with Urie's Fish Fry, though it's owned by the same family, this younger sibling sports more modern quarters in Urie's Motel and the old-line menu is heavy on the prime rib and steaks. The Pegleg Lounge (God help us) features late-night snacks and happy hour—and everyone in town seems to show up. Hours are seasonal.

Ventura's Greenhouse $23

106 S. Benson Ave., Margate (609) 822-0140
next to Lucy the Elephant at the Jersey Shore

Affectionately known as "Greenie" to its fans, this beach-convenient, family-friendly Italian sports the "best pizza on the coast" (note the "great spinach" pies), along with a broad menu heavy on the hoagies, burgers, salads. There's an outdoor deck in season and an even more casual downstairs cafe that offers up nightly specials year-round, including all-you-can eat mussels twice a week. Watch out for seasonal hours.

Viana's $23

Whitehorse Rd., Voorhees (609) 770-0824
bet. Rt. 561 & Whitehorse Pk. in So. Jersey

Known for homemade pastas and fresh fish, Viana's strikes our reviewers as a "very nice" place for good Italian food in the Voorhees area. Relaxed, homey atmosphere and moderate prices make this one to try.

 = Superior = Excellent = Very Good

Viennese Cafe

$25

1442 Rt. 70 E., Cherry Hill (609) 795-0172 (at Rt. 295 in So. Jersey)
"Surprisingly good food" and "friendly service" have attracted a loyal following at this charming, family-oriented Country French-cum-Northern Italian cafe that offers "loads of freebies" and terrific homemade desserts. The "European cuisine" is "very inexpensive," according to our Reporters, especially when you consider the "huge portions." There's even a piano bar for late-night "fun."

Vitarelli's

$18

1250 Kings Hwy N., Cherry Hill (609) 429-9088
Rt. 70 in So. Jersey
There is a good, solid feel at this Cherry Hill Neighborhood Italian restaurant. It's family-style, and while they aren't making culinary history in the kitchen, there's something to be said for the old, traditional standbys. Don't be scared by the room rating: it's your cue to dress casually and bring the kids. Unfortunately, there's no separate smoking section. Byo.

Washington Inn

$39

801 Washington St., Cape May (609) 884-5697
at Jefferson at the Jersey Shore
"The best wine list anywhere" is just one of the draws at this "romantic," "beautiful" Cape May Continental that wins plenty of plaudits from its fans. The "charming old inn atmosphere" (try to snag a table on the "enclosed porch") is the perfect setting for "gracious" service and "excellent" food that's "always consistent." Christmas is a particularly wonderful time to visit, when the inn puts on an authentic Dickens dinner complete with Dickensian food and actors. No matter when you come, however, "make reservations way in advance."

Waterfront

$27

998 Bay Ave., Somers Point (609) 653-0099
at the Jersey Shore
"There's no gourmet at the Waterfront," but the "utilitarian" American-trendy food is hardly the point of this huge, hoppin' "pick-up scene" that offers a "great" view of the bay and an open-air bar featuring live music seven nights a week in season. "Typical shore fare," sure, but "when it's time to leave the shore and you're feeling a little low, this place will pick you right up."

Waters Edge

$42

Beach & Pittsburgh Aves., Cape May (609) 884-1717
at the Jersey Shore
One of the few Cape May restaurants with an ocean view, chef-owner Neil Elsohn's creative American in an unlikely motel-side location delivers up "spectacular" imaginative cuisine in sleek comfortable quarters at the end of the beach. The "nice Sunday breakfast outside" in the summer is a wonderful touch at this well-regarded spot that has eluded the crowds and crush of in-town Cape May.

FOOD ROOM STAFF COST

White House Sub Shop

$10

2301 Arctic Ave., Atlantic City (609) 345-1564
at Mississippi Ave. at the Jersey Shore

"The best hoagie, bar none" is yours for the asking (and a couple of bucks) at this Formica-and celebrity-photo-intensive sandwich shop that has been dishing out "rude service" and "the best subs you can get" since 1946. The "best tuna sub on the East Coast" is second only to the "best cheesesteak in the world," thanks to the "best-tasting rolls" around. "Why can't the hoagies in Philadelphia be like the White House Hoagies?" Perhaps "they should franchise."

Wild Orchid

$30

127 Ark Rd., Larchmont Shopping Ctr., Mt. Laurel (609) 273-0002
at Rt. 38 in So. Jersey

A "top-rated" spot in South Jersey, this "excellent" chef-owned cafe offers Glen Feller's "consistently innovative and wonderful" seasonal American cuisine (including "great breads," "superb sauces," the "best steak" and soups, and "knockout desserts"). The "interesting" menu is complemented by a well-trained staff who know how to serve a "fabulous meal." The only complaint seems to be about the less-than-wow storefront decor, but otherwise, Wild Orchid is "highly recommended." BYOB, and save room for the "chocolate macadamia brownies."

Windrift

$27

79th St. & Beach, Avalon (609) 368-5761 (at the Jersey Shore)

The "beach location" is "perfect for brunch" or the "pick-up" scene at happy hour, especially if you're in the mood for a "cold beer on a hot day" in Avalon. Though there's no view of the ocean, some of the dining rooms sit right on the dunes, so it stands to reason that there'd be lots of seafood on the menu. Fans enthuse about the "great" broiled crab cakes and sauteed crabmeat, and the "consistently good" staff gets a nod, too. P.S. Closed in winter.

Zagara's

$20

501 Rt. 73 S., Towne Place at Marlton, Marlton (609) 983-5700
at Brick Rd. in So. Jersey

"The best gourmet grocery" in the area wows our reviewers with an "eye-boggling selection" of high-quality food, from the "wonderful Italian delicacies" and prepared foods to "great bread, fresh produce, and salad bar." Sure, it's mobbed on weekends, but the "extraordinary" assortment of "marvelous" stuff at this "upscale market" makes it "one of the all-time-great places to stop" for a while. No wonder so many folks say they "couldn't live without it."

Delaware

Amalfi

$32

3801 Kennett Pk., Greenville (302) 655-7719 at Buck Rd.
This upscale Greenville Italian gets very good grades for a menu highlighted by homemade pasta and seafood dishes (cioppino, fish stew in red sauce, is a specialty). Service needs a little work and the room is small, "very close" for some, "cozy" for others, so reservations are essential.

Back Burner

$32

Old Lancaster Pk., Hockessin Corner, Hockessin (302) 239-2314
"It's odd," writes one reviewer, "to find a great place in such an out-of-the-way area." But find it they do, and they also find one of the top 20 best spots for food in our poll. The "excellent American food" is "a perennial favorite," from the Black Angus strip steak to their famous pumpkin mushroom soup. The burners themselves are on display, as the kitchen is open to the restaurant, contributing to the "noisy" room. In sum, our voters say it is "excellent and special."

Bangkok House

$22

104 N. Union St., Wilm. (302) 654-8555 bet. Lancaster Pk. & 2nd St.
Family owned, this storefront Thai has become a fixture in the Wilmington scene after eight years of service. The decor, above average for an ethnic place, is authentic Thai, as are the duck dishes, combination salads and curry dishes. A standout of the "great food" is the "best pad Thai," though crispy sprouts and peanutty sate run close seconds.

Blue Moon

35 Baltimore Ave., Rehoboth Beach (302) 227-6515 (at 1st St.)
This New American helped spark Rehoboth's restaurant revolution in the '80s, and its pull has never waned, thanks to flights of fancy like the moon pie, filled with homemade ice cream and topped with baked meringue. Voters find the bold decor and cutting-edge cuisine "delightful" and say it's "still the nicest gay spot in Rehoboth."

Brandywine Room at the Hotel du Pont

$45

11th & Market Sts., Hotel duPont, Wilmington (302) 594-3156
Though less formal than the hotel's Green Room, the Brandywine room—with its rich walnut paneling and impressive collection of original art by three generations of Wyeths—is still one of the fanciest dining rooms in Wilmington. The American-Continental menu is long on beef and seafood, and the service a dream. Reservations essential.

Buckley's Tavern

$25

5812 Kennett Pk., Centreville (302) 656-9776
Dine in the tavern, the more formal dining room or on the rooftop deck at this venerable Regional American in Centreville, close to Winterthur Museum and Longwood Gardens. The tavern, a "big local bar scene hangout," gets noisy. The food earns solid if unspectacular scores (the crab cakes win raves), not bad considering the mid-level prices. A treat for wine-lovers: You can choose from the wine list or browse in an adjoining wine shop, buy a bottle and bring it to your table—without paying a restaurant markup or corkage fee.

FOOD ROOM STAFF COST

Carucci

$46

504 Greenhill Ave., Wawaset Plaza, Wilmington (302) 654-2333

This small, contemporary Italian sleeper in Wilmington is notable for its "unique, stylish" decor, 25 wines by the glass and prize-winning opera singers who double as waiters. But it gets its highest marks for cuisine, especially from those who find the staff's vocalizing "a pain."

Charcoal Pit

$11

Fox Run Shopping Ctr., Bear (302) 834-3000
2600 Concord Pk., Wilmington (302) 478-2165
5200 Pike Creek Ctr. Blvd., Wilmington (302) 999-7483

A '50s North Wilmington burger joint that has survived into the '90s by concentrating on "tasty, inexpensive steak sandwiches and "unbeatable" burgers. Some voters say "the quality has gone down" since the opening of branches in the western suburbs.

Chili's

$16

425 Stanton-Christiana Rd., Newark (302) 738-6355

Chili's scores look unimpressive until they're stacked up against similar chains. While some voters have had "awful" experiences, many say it's "a great place to take the kids—$1 per!" The food isn't great, but it's "better than you'd expect," and "children and parents can both enjoy it and be comfortable."

Columbus Inn

$33

2216 Pennsylvania Ave., Wilmington (302) 571-1492 at Woodlawn

This Wilmington American-Continental sometimes explores new trends, but customers always return to old beef and seafood favorites. Voters say it's a "good business lunch spot" and that the food, while sometimes "so-so," is "improving under a new chef." Its highest grades are for the 18th-century building's ambiance, which is supplemented by piano music on weekends.

Constantinou's House of Beef

$32

1616 Delaware Ave., Wilmington (302) 652-0653
bet. DuPont & Clayton Sts.

The name indicates the specialty at this American in Wilmington's Trolley Square—big cuts of beef, grilled on an open hearth. The restaurant offers lots of tableside preparations and flaming desserts, and though voters aren't impressed with the general quality of the service, they hope the new owners will change that.

DiNardo's

$25

405 N. Lincoln St., Wilmington (302) 656-3685
bet 4th & 5th Sts.

The strengths and weaknesses of this crab house in Wilmington's Little Italy mirror those at the Philadelphia branch—"best crabs in the world" (or at least "best crabs in the area") in a no-frills atmosphere (if you're famous enough, they'll ask you to sign the wall). Romac Reporters who've been to both say this is "better than the one in Philly."

 = Superior = Excellent = Very Good

Green Room at the Hotel du Pont

$44

11th. & Market Sts., Hotel du Pont, Wilmington (302) 594-3154

Voters are wowed by the opulent, formal French dining room in downtown Wilmington's landmark hotel, where "the atmosphere and service can't be duplicated." A mostly older crowd appreciates the pre-WWI elegance—massive chandeliers dangle from a vaulted, coffered ceiling decorated with gold leaf—and can afford "food that's worth every expensive penny." The staff gets excellent ratings and brunch is "a world-class experience" at what many call "the best room in the area."

Griglia Toscana

$35

1412 N. Du Pont St., Rockford Shops, Wilmington (302) 654-8001
bet. Delaware Ave. & 14th St.

Romac reporters rave about the "great Italian menu," "outstanding pasta" at this upscale neighborhood bistro in Wilmington where everything is made from scratch. The large, open room, featuring an open kitchen and wood-burning pizza oven at one end, has a cosmopolitan feel more popular with younger voters, but all commend the fresh salads, "great grilled selection" and, first and foremost, the pasta. They also like the mid-range prices. Even with reservations, which are essential, there's sometimes a wait for a table.

Grotto Pizza

$13

Rt. 202, Fairfax Shopping Ctr., Wilmington (302) 888-2222
Main St., Newark (302) 369-2200
Rt. 202, Brandywine Commons, Wilmington (302) 479-8300

If you want to get to all of the top 10 pizza places in the poll, you'll have to go to Wilmington to this little spot on Route 202. "Too bad it's so far away," writes onc Philadelphian, but Wilmingtonians happily rejoice in that fact, calling it the "best pizza in town." The room and staff are better than a lot of Philly pie joints, though they do their best business with delivery and takeout.

Harry's Savoy Grill

$28

2020 Naamans Rd., Wilmington (302) 475-3000 (bet. Marsh & Foulk)

This North Wilmington American's success can be traced to beef and seafood that get very good marks at relatively low prices. The "beautiful English country interiors" captivate some, but voters rate the ambiance and service below the food. A "great bar" features a wide choice of microbrews and single-malt scotches. Though a kids' menu is offered, the highest scores come from the over-40 set. The brunch also comes highly recommended.

Italian Bistro

$22

Christiana Mall, Newark (302) 366-8566

"Surprisingly good," writes one voter. Well, creativity would be a surprise from an Italian Bistro with this name. "A great place for all," meaning families, say reviewers, though they are more inclined to talk about this mini-chain's more exotic locations, like "in the Ocean Mall in Atlantic City." The "nice bar" has an above-average selection of wines by the glass, and the pastries are also recommended. No reservations taken.

FOOD ROOM STAFF COST

Jake's Hamburgers

VOTE

1100 Ogletown Rd., Newark (302) 737-1118
at Marrows Rd.

Picnic tables, no bathrooms, just basic burgers cooked on a griddle—this burger joint on the edge of college-town Newark is popular with a young crowd as a sort of anti-McDonald's.

La La Land

VOTE

22 Wilmington Ave., Rehoboth Beach (302) 227-3887 at the Ocean blk.

Voters love this seasonal Rehoboth Eclectic whether they're dining inside the Victorian cottages or amid the bamboo on the patio. Chef David Keener's "food is passionate," both in flavor and "very artistic presentation," attracting a clientele as eclectic as the California-style menu.

Michele's

VOTE

1828 W. 11th St., Wilmington (302) 655-8554
bet. Lincoln & Scott

This Continental fills two floors of a row house on the edge of Wilmington's Little Italy—the formal Victorian upstairs room bans smoking, the more urbane downstairs allows it. The menu mixes French and Italian dishes with a dash of modern presentation.

Mirage

$29

100 Elkton Rd., Newark (302) 453-1711
at Main St.

Voters still give this Newark New American's "creative food" and "superb presentation" good marks, and the staff rates even higher, but a few longtime customers say they've been disappointed lately. With the University of Delaware in town, the vegetarian entrees are unusually inspired. Prices are reasonable.

Shipley Grill

$27

913 Shipley Rd , Historic Boines Building, Wilmington
(302) 652-7797 (1/2 block behind Hotel DuPont)

The food is the big draw at this Wilmington New American, which scores significantly higher among voters in the 31-45 group; older Romac Reporters say the one-time tavern is a "boring room." "Great waitstaff" makes the Shipley a favorite both before and after performances at the nearby Playhouse and Grand Opera House.

Silk Purse & Sow's Ear

$40

1307 N. Scott St., Wilmington (302) 654-7666
at Pennsylvania Ave.

These Wilmington Eclectics have separate entrances but the same kitchen. The upstairs Sow's Ear, begun as a bistro alternative to the formal Silk Purse, has surpassed it in popularity, but many voters feel the "upstairs and downstairs are equally neat." The "imaginative menu" mixes French and Italian dishes with Pacific Rim and Southwestern touches for a meal that's "expensive but worth it."

 = Superior = Excellent = Very Good

Sydney's Side Street

$34

25 Christian St., Rehoboth Beach (302) 227-1339

This Rehoboth Regional American tilts toward New Orleans-style cuisine, and offers jazz and blues to match Thursday through Sunday in season. The off-season pairing is even more profound—gospel music with Sunday brunch. Voters also "love the grazing room," where they can sample a wider variety of smaller portions.

Terrace at Greenhill

$21

800 N. Dupont Rd., Wilmington (302) 575-1990 (at Lancaster Ave.)

The food is solid, but the "wonderful view of the downtown Wilmington skyline" is spectacular at this Regional American overlooking the Porky Oliver golf course. Just as many cite the "reasonable" prices, which also makes it a popular business lunch spot.

Tiffin

$32

1210 N. Market St., Wilmington (302) 571-1133 (bet. 12th & 13th)

This downtown Wilmington spot is a favorite with the business crowd for its "smart, distinctive" modern American menu in a "nice contemporary atmosphere"—dining rooms in two 19th century brick buildings look out on a plant-filled atrium between them, so it "feels like you're eating in a courtyard."

Trevi

$25

3100 Naamans Rd., The Shoppes at Naamans, Wilmington (302) 478-7434 (Shipley Rd. & Rt. 202)

This North Wilmington Italian exudes old-world charm and atmosphere despite its shopping-center location, especially on Wednesdays and Sundays, when an accordion player strolls the rooms accompanied by a tenor (the owner's father). Whatever night you go, you'll find "good quality at a good price."

Vincente's

$38

1601 Concord Pk., Independence Mall, Wilmington (302) 652-9387

This upscale Italian recently relocated from Wilmington's Little Italy to its northern suburbs, putting the room rating in doubt. Reviewers tend to judge the food either superb or so-so, but the service really shines, reflecting maitre d' Vincent Mancari's flamboyant tableside presentations of Caesar salad and flaming desserts.

INDEXES:

CUISINE TYPES

NEIGHBORHOODS

FEATURES

Cuisine Types

BBQ

Belgian

Brazilian

Burmese

Cajun/Creole

Californian

Caribbean

Cheesesteaks, Hoagies, etc.

Crabs

Deli

Desserts

Eclectic

Philadelphia Neighborhoods

Philadelphia Suburbs and Beyond

New Jersey

Delaware

Features

Brunch

food rating=very good or better

Catering

food rating=very good or better

Child-friendly

Credit Cards Not Taken

Dancing

Delivery

food rating=very good or better

Dessert a Specialty

food rating=very good or better

Dim Sum

Early Bird Specials

food rating=very good or better

Hospital Health Menu

Hotel Dining

food rating=very good or better

Inn Dining

food rating=very good or better

Jacket/Tie Required

Outdoor Dining

Pre-Theater Menu

food rating=very good or better

Prix Fixe Dinner

food rating=very good or better

Saturday Lunch, Center City

food rating=very good or better

Smoking Not Permitted

Tea (English Afternoon Tea)

Wheelchair Access

We conducted a separate phone survey to create this list. Each restaurant has to meet four criteria. First, there is no step at the entrance. Second, there is no step on the way to the restroom. Third, the restroom is large enough for a wheelchair to access the toilet. Fourth, there is a handrail bolted to the wall next to the toilet. Please call ahead to make certain the restaurant's facilities meet your needs.

THE ROMAC REPORT BUSINESS EDITION

Give the Romac Report

- ***Before the holidays;***
- ***At the close of a deal;***
- ***At the promotion of a new product or service;***
- ***Before a meeting or conference.***

Your company's name and/or message imprinted in gold leaf on the cover

For more information, call (610) 519-0600

Order Form

QUANTITY	COST
5,000 or more	$6.95
2,500 to 4,999	7.45
1,000 to 2,499	7.95
500 to 999	8.95
250 to 499	9.95
100 to 249	11.95
50 to 99	12.95
25 to 49	13.95

Custom die stamp $50
Mailing boxes. . . . . $.50

**Imprint charge, shipping and handling included.
Supply camera ready to avoid add'l setup charge.**

NAME ____________________

COMPANY NAME ____________________

POSITION ____________________

STREET ADDRESS ____________________

CITY, STATE ZIP ____________________

PHONE ____________ FAX ____________

☐ **Please send me**

_________ copies
@ _________ ea
_________ subtotal
+ $50 custom stamp
+ 6% _________ sales tax
_________ **total**

☐ **Please send more information about the Romac Report Business Edition**

ROMAC

REPORT

PLACE
STAMP
HERE

ROMAC REPORT

Romac Report Business Edition
P.O. Box 328
Villanova, PA 19085